Evidence-based Dentistry:
Managing Information for Better Practice

Quintessentials of Dental Practice – 41
Clinical Practice – 7

Evidence-based Dentistry:
Managing Information for Better Practice

By

**Derek Richards, Jan Clarkson,
Debora Matthews and Richard Niederman**

Editor-in-Chief: Nairn H F Wilson
Editor Clinical Practice: Nairn H F Wilson

Quintessence Publishing Co. Ltd.
London, Berlin, Chicago, Paris, Milan, Barcelona, Istanbul,
São Paulo, Tokyo, New Delhi, Moscow, Prague, Warsaw

British Library Cataloguing in Publication Data

Evidence-based dentistry: managing information for better practice.
- (Quintessentials of dental practice; v. 41)
1. Evidence-based dentistry
I. Richards, Derek
617.6

ISBN-13: 9781850971269

ISBN-13: 978-1-85097-126-9

Foreword

You must have come across the term "evidence-based dentistry" (EBD). But do you really understand it, are you practising it and, if not, can you hand-on-heart say that your clinical decisions and treatments are best for your patients? *Evidence-based Dentistry: Managing Information for Better Practice* adds yet another dimension to the *Quintessentials of Dental Practice* series. The volume provides a valuable introduction to EBD, including guidance as to how to apply this approach to your clinical practice. The concepts underpinning the evidence-based approach to clinical decision-making and treatment provision are not new; however, the move to achieving widespread application of the approach is relatively recent. If you are not part of this movement, or need to know more about the application of the approach, then this book will be a valuable acquisition. As has come to be expected of all *Quintessential* volumes, this book is a carefully crafted, easy to read, well-illustrated text, including a wealth of sound advice and practical guidance of immediate practical relevance – a key to many benefits to your patients and practice, let alone a portal to enhanced professional fulfilment.

Congratulations to the author and contributors for a job well done – another jewel in the *Quintessentials'* treasure-trove.

Nairn Wilson
Editor-in-Chief

Preface

When talking to practitioners about evidence-based dentistry (EBD) there are a number of questions that are commonly raised:

- Is EBD new?
- Would I need to change my practice to be evidence-based?
- Could EBD save me time and money?
- Would my patients benefit from EBD?
- Is it easy?
- Is it really different from what I do now?
- Do I need to understand statistics?

Practitioners strive day to day to do their best for their patients and in doing so make many decisions on how to treat them. The influences on this decision-making process are many and varied.

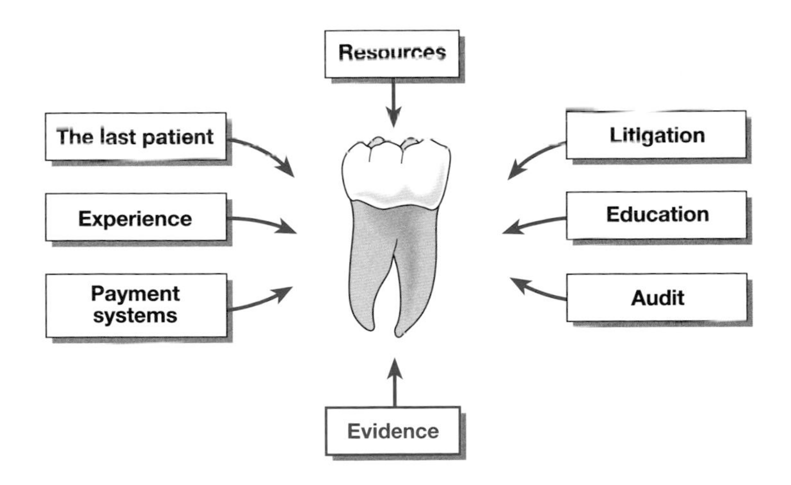

Evidence is just one of these influences, but an important one. The term evidence-based dentistry was introduced to the dental world in 1994 (see Evidence-Based Medicine Working Group, 1994). Now as then, when dentists are asked, they say their practice is based on evidence. However, when the evidence has been reviewed for some of the most frequently performed techniques, the lack of quality evidence is apparent. Conversely, there are some simple procedures where evidence of benefit exists and yet they are not routinely performed.

This book aims to provide both undergraduates and postgraduates of all ages with an introduction to EBD and the techniques with which to apply it in practice, and in the process answer the questions posed above.

Reference

Evidence-Based Medicine Working Group. Evidence-based health care: a new approach to teaching the practice of health care. J Dent Educ 1994;58(8):648–653.

Acknowledgements

The authors are indebted to the Cochrane Oral Health Group and the following individuals and publishers who have allowed us to reproduce their material, which has made this book possible: Bazian (Box 4-1), The Public Health Resource Unit, Oxford, for the CASP worksheets (Figs 5-3, 8-2, 9-2 and 10-1), the *Journal of Contemporary Dental Practice* (Box 6-1), Nature Publishing (Fig 9-1) and permission to use the glossary from the *Evidence-based Dentistry Journal*, Dr Amanda Burls for permission to use the material presented in Fig 8-5, Dr Andy Hall and Nicola Innes for clinical images for senarios A, B, D and E.

We would like to thank Dr Janet Harris for her comments on the qualitative studies chapter and we are also indebted to Alison Richards and Diane Lynas for checking and proofreading the manuscript.

Contents

Chapter 1

Introduction

Aim

The aim of this chapter is to define evidence-based dentistry and outline the five-stage evidence-based method.

Outcome

After completing this chapter readers will be familiar with the definition of evidence based dentistry and the five stages.

What is Evidence-based Dentistry (EBD)?

Evidence-based dentistry is a method for rapidly aggregating, distilling and implementing the best evidence in clinical practice (Sackett et al., 1996; Straus et al., 2005). Successfully accomplishing this requires the integration of:

- the best clinical evidence
- clinical judgement, together with
- patient values and circumstances, to improve healthcare (Fig 1-1).

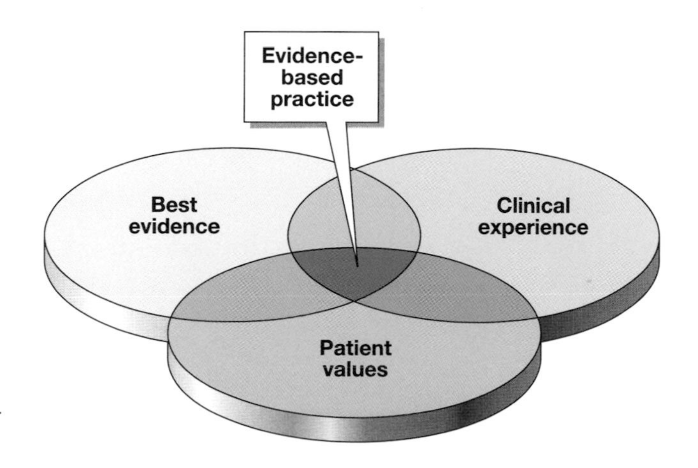

Fig 1-1 Evidence-based practice.

Delegates at the second international conference of evidence-based healthcare teachers in Sicily discussed the need for a clear definition of what constitutes evidence-based practice (EBP), what skills are needed to practise in an evidence-based manner and a curriculum that outlines the minimum requirements for training health professionals in EBP. They produced the Sicily consensus statement on evidence-based practice (see Dawes et al., 2005).

Is EBD New?

The ideas associated with the evidence-based approach have been around a long time. In the second edition of their textbook, Sackett et al. (2000) linked their ideas with post-revolutionary Paris, while Sir Iain Chalmers, in a lecture to celebrate International Clinical Trials Day in 2006 (see Chalmers, 2006), suggested origins in ancient China or the Middle East.

This delay in uptake of the most effective treatments was one of the driving forces behind the development of the evidence-based approach to healthcare. This current trend developed from a group based in McMaster University in Canada who introduced the term evidence-based medicine in 1992.

Dentists will recognise the picture of bleeding gums (Fig 1-2). Scurvy, one of its more unusual causes, is a good example of an evidential approach and of the challenges in getting evidence-based treatments adopted as common practice (Box 1-1).

Best Evidence

Early in the development of EBD the approach was criticised for focusing on evidence from randomised controlled trials and systematic reviews of

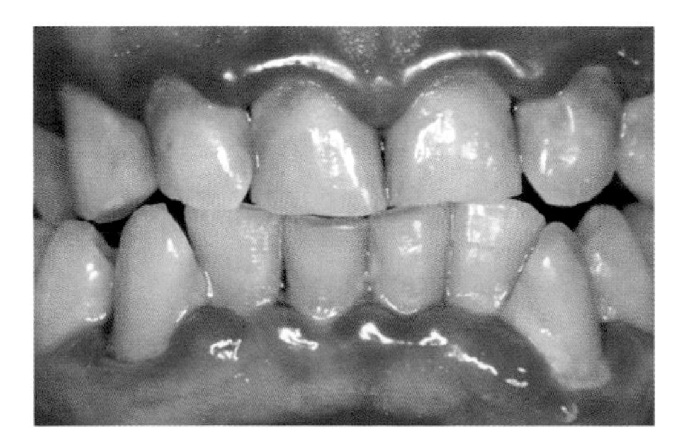

Fig 1-2 Periodontal disease.

Box 1-1 **James Lind and scurvy**

Lind, in his treatise of the scurvy (Lind, 1753), summarises his trial conducted on 12 patients:

"*On 20th May 1747, I took twelve patients in the scurvy, on board the Salisbury at sea. Their cases were as similar as I could have them. They all in general had putrid gums, the spots and lassitude, with weakness of their knees. They lay together in one place, being a proper apartment for the sick in the fore-hold; and had one diet common to all.*"

Two sailors were allocated to each of:

- "*a quart of cyder daily*
- *25 gutts of elixir vitriol thrice daily*
- *2 spoonfuls of vinegar thrice daily*
- *half a pint of sea water daily*
- *two oranges and a lemon daily*
- *the bigness of a nutmeg thrice daily.*"

As we know, those on fresh fruit did best but, despite presenting this study together with a systematic review of the available evidence in his 1753 treatise, it was not until 1795 that the Royal Navy ordered ships to carry supplies of lemons! This is not an uncommon experience, with effective treatments taking many years to get into widespread use.

evidence. There has been a shift in this position, with the clear view that what is required is evidence from the most appropriate study design to answer the clinical question being posed (Table 1-1).

Early systematic reviews in healthcare were focused on randomised controlled trials (RCTs) but the past decade has seen development of systematic review methodology for a range of study designs. The availability of high-quality systematic reviews is increasing through the work of groups like the Cochrane and Campbell Collaborations and increased use of these reviews will improve the quality of evidence available for decision-making. The availability of these reviews means that information about effective treatment is more readily available; this can bring benefit to patients and potentially save time and money by providing effective treatments and abandoning ineffective ones.

Table 1-1 **Study designs to answer clinical questions**

	Type of research				
	Qualitative	**Case-control**	**Cohort**	**RCT**	**Systematic review**
Diagnosis			✓	✓✓	✓✓✓
Treatment			✓	✓✓	✓✓✓
Screening				✓✓	✓✓✓
Service delivery	✓	✓	✓	✓✓	✓✓✓
Safety				✓✓	✓✓✓
Acceptability				✓✓	✓✓✓
Quality	✓	✓	✓		✓✓✓

Adapted from Muir Gray JA. Evidence-based health care: how to make health policy and management decisions. London: Churchill Livingstone, 1997.

Clinical Expertise

Clinical expertise is a key element and this can and will vary significantly. As with most things in life, experience in providing one type of treatment or using certain materials, procedures or equipment will vary. In addition, while you may have experience of using particular materials, procedures or equipment, they may not always be available in every circumstance. It is for these reasons that clinical experience is an important element in making evidence-based decisions.

Patient Values

Patients' values play a crucial role in evidence-based practice, but articulating these values is a challenge for some of them. It is also important to recognise that there are three competing value systems for the three stakeholders involved in clinical decisions (the patient, the dentist, and the third-party payer – be it the state or an insurer). Recognising this, and engaging patients in simultaneous discussion about values, evidence and clinical judgement will help improve the quality of the provided care.

Why an Evidence-based Approach?

The main reason to implement EBD is to improve the quality of care. The introduction of clinical audit and peer review and the move towards lifelong learning have been drivers for change within healthcare. They have been coupled with an increasing focus on the quality and consistency of healthcare provision and a desire to avoid unnecessary treatment.

Another factor has been the increasing involvement of patients in healthcare decision-making. This has been welcomed by the profession for the most part. The driver for this (and one of the main drivers for the introduction of EBD) is the enormous amount of information that is available today. This is in the form of books, journals and the internet.

The almost ubiquitous availability of the internet and general ease of access makes this both a useful and a powerful tool. For example, if you type the word "dental" into the search engine Google, you get about 226,000,000 hits: 4,100,000 for "caries" and 8,520,000 for "dental implants".

What Is an Evidence-based Approach?

Essentially, EBP is a set of methods for rapidly aggregating, distilling and implementing the best clinical information in clinical practice. The approach consists of five steps (the 5 As). Each stage has been subjected to trials of teaching effectiveness.

The evidence-based method

1. Asking answerable questions	(ASK)
2. Searching for the best evidence	(ACQUIRE)
3. Critically appraising the evidence	(APPRAISE)
4. Applying the evidence	(APPLY)
5. Evaluating the outcome	(ASSESS)

While most clinicians will not engage in developing evidence, they can relatively easily become effective users of evidence. This book provides an introduction to EBP and the techniques with which to apply it to your practice.

However, it should be emphasised that EBP is an active problem-based approach to acquiring and developing knowledge that needs to be practised. It is therefore best learned and appreciated in small group workshops and active participation.

Key Points

Evidence-based practice:

- is a structured approach for clinical decision-making
- assists the practitioner in finding, distilling, and applying the best evidence in clinical practice
- manages the problem of information overload and uncertainty.

References

Chalmers I (ed.) Evolution of Fair Tests of Medical Treatments: Celebrating International Clinical Trials Day – an International Story. James Lind Library, 2006, Abu Bakr Muhammad ibn Zakariyya al-Razi (Rhazes), 865–925.

Dawes M et al. Sicily statement on evidence-based practice. BMC Med Educ 2005;5:1.

Lind J. A treatise of the scurvy. In three parts. Containing an inquiry into the nature, causes and cure, of that disease. Together with a critical and chronological view of what has been published on the subject. Printed by Sands, Murray and Cochran for A Kincaid and A Donaldson: Edinburgh, 1753.

Sackett DL, Rosenberg WM, Gray JA, Haynes RB, Richardson WS. Evidence based medicine: what it is and what it isn't. Br Med J 1996;312(7023):71–72.

Sackett DL, Straus SE, Richardson WS, Rosenberg W, Haynes RB. Evidence-based Medicine: How to Practise and Teach EBM. 2nd edn. Edinburgh: Churchill Livingstone, 2000.

Straus SE, Richardson WS, Glasziou P, Haynes RB. Evidence-based Medicine: How to Practise and Teach EBM. 3rd edn. Edinburgh: Churchill Livingstone, 2005.

Chapter 2
Finding Answers

Aim

This chapter outlines a hierarchy of evidence sources to answer clinical problems.

Outcome

After completing this chapter readers will be able to describe a hierarchy of sources to find the best available evidence.

Hierarchy of Evidence

Time is at a premium for most practitioners and the majority will want to find answers to their clinical problems quickly and simply. While having a clear question puts you on the right track we know that it is answers that practitioners want. In terms of where best to find answers of high quality, a clear hierarchy can be described:

1. Evidence-based clinical guidelines
2. Cochrane systematic reviews
3. Systematic reviews
4. Studies.

This hierarchy is a simplification based on the levels of evidence tables produced by a range of groups. One of the most detailed of these is available from the Centre for Evidence-Based Medicine website at: www.cebm.net/index.aspx?o=1025.

The hierarchy should be thought of as a distillation or filtering process (Fig 2-1) as Cochrane and other systematic reviews are derived from existing studies and evidence-based guidelines are a synthesis of Cochrane reviews, systematic reviews and studies.

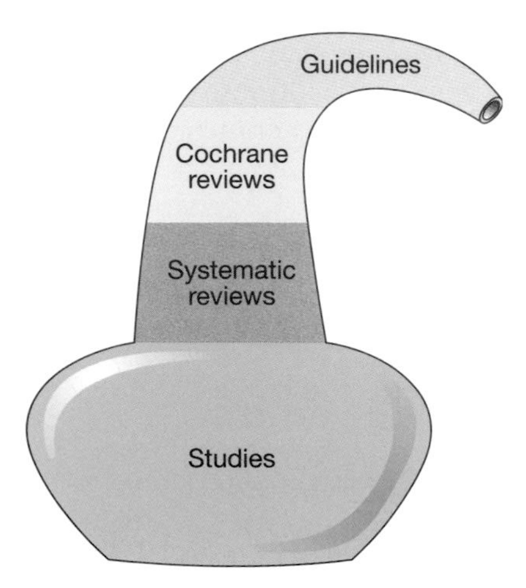

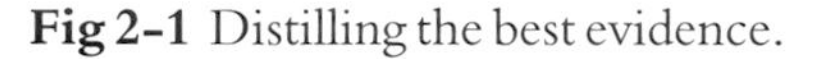
Fig 2-1 Distilling the best evidence.

Evidence-based Guidelines

In terms of application of evidence to clinical practice, evidence-based practice guidelines are the best place to start for most practitioners. The development of clinical practice guidelines based on evidence in dentistry is relatively new. Although a number of organisations have produced parameters and standards of care and expert-derived or consensus-based guidelines, there are very few published, peer-reviewed, evidence-based clinical practice guidelines validated by practising dentists.

The best guidelines use an evidence-based process to systematically assemble, organise and synthesise the best available evidence from clinical research. Ideally, these are based on *systematic reviews* of the literature, which use rigorous and explicit methods to search for and critically appraise the entire body of clinical research evidence related to the question. The methodology is well documented, allowing anyone (who wishes to do so) to replicate the results. This evidence is then integrated with clinical expertise from a number of practitioners and patients to develop workable clinical recommendations. Each guideline is intended for use in *specific* conditions or circumstances. The clinician is expected to take into account each patient's history and preferences, together with their own clinical experience and judgement, when applying a guideline.

A major advantage of guidelines is that they save the clinician several steps when trying to solve a clinical dilemma. They serve to "translate" evidence from clinical research into language easily understood by clinicians, i.e. they have already carried out the first three of our 5 As – Ask, Acquire, Appraise, Apply and Assess. Many guidelines also provide a patient version as well, which can serve to assist communications between clinicians and patients.

Evidence-based guidelines can be found at the websites given in Table 2-1.

Cochrane Systematic Reviews

Cochrane systematic reviews are prepared by the Cochrane Collaboration (see page 41) and published in the Cochrane Library (see page 115). These reviews are prepared using well-defined systematic methods to limit bias (systematic errors) and reduce chance effects (Box 2-1), thus providing more reliable results from which to draw conclusions and make decisions.

Table 2-1 **URLs for evidence-based guideline development groups in oral health**

Guideline development programmes		
USA	National Guideline Clearinghouse	www.guideline.gov
England	National Institute of Clinical Excellence (NICE), NHS	www.nice.org.uk
	Royal College of Surgeons of England	www.rcseng.ac.uk/fds/clinical_guidelines
Scotland	Scottish Intercollegiate Network (SIGN)	www.sign.ac.uk
	Scottish Dental Clinical Effectiveness Programme (SDCEP)	www.scottishdental.org/cep
Sweden	Swedish Council on Technology Assessment in Health Care (SBU)	www.sbu.se/www/index.asp

Box 2-1 **Systematic reviews**

A review which strives to identify, appraise and summarise all relevant evidence on a topic comprehensively, according to agreed criteria. The key elements in a systematic review are to:

- specify objectives
- report all relevant primary studies
- assess methodological quality
- identify common definitions for outcomes
- extract estimates of outcomes
- meta-analyse where appropriate
- provide a narrative summary where data are sparse or of too low a quality
- explore robustness of results
- clearly present key aspects
- appraise methodological limitations of primary studies and systematically review.

During the 1970s and 1980s, psychologists and social scientists had drawn attention to the systematic steps needed to minimise bias and random errors in reviews of research (see Light and Smith, 1971; Glass, 1976; Rosenthal, 1978; Jackson, 1980; Cooper, 1982). However, it was not until the late 1980s that people drew attention to the poor scientific quality of healthcare review articles (see Mulrow, 1987; Yusuf et al., 1987; Oxman and Guyatt, 1988).

Many of these reviews were "narrative" – that is, they were often written by a single topic expert based on his or her understanding of the literature. The literature may be searched but this is likely to be biased to support the ideas of the reviewer. This is not done deliberately, but nonetheless, rarely is any methodology described so the process is reproducible. This means that the reader is unable to check the assumptions of the authors or replicate the process.

Cochrane reviews follow a clear methodology described in Higgins and Green's (2006) extensive handbook, a rigorous peer review process and a commitment for them to be updated regularly which distinguishes them from other systematic reviews. The key differences between systematic reviews and narrative reviews are outlined in Table 2-2.

Table 2-2 **Key differences between narrative and systematic reviews**

Feature	Narrative review	Systematic review
Question	Broad scope	Focused
Sources and search	Not usually specified	Comprehensive and explicit
Appraisal	Variable	Rigorous
Synthesis	Often qualitative summary	Quantitative summary
Inferences	Sometimes evidence-based	Usually evidence-based

Systematic Reviews

Since the development of systematic review methodologies (Cochrane Methodology – see Higgins and Green, 2006; Centre for Reviews and Dissemination – see Khan et al., 2001), an increasing number of systematic reviews are becoming available. There are a number of differences between Cochrane and non-Cochrane systematic reviews. As noted above, the quality of peer review in Cochrane reviews is much more robust than with others (see Olsen et al., 2001). They strive for greater transparency and are updated when relevant new evidence is available. However, the majority of Cochrane reviews are conducted on randomised controlled trials. With the emergence of standards for the reporting of systematic reviews in a range of areas (Table 2-3), other systematic reviews are emerging that apply to more than just randomised trials.

Studies

If there are no evidence-based guidelines or systematic reviews available, you need to be able to find one or more individual studies to be able to answer the relevant clinical questions. The main types of studies you would need to answer these questions are outlined in Table 2-4.

One problem with individual studies is that, despite the recent increase in the number of practice-based research networks, the majority of studies are conducted in academic environments on highly selected patients. This can

Table 2-3 **Standards for the reporting of systematic reviews**

Standard	Description	Website
QUOROM statement	Improving the quality of reports of meta-analyses of randomised controlled trials	www.consort-statement.org/index.aspx?o=1065
MOOSE proposals	Proposal for reporting meta-analysis of observational studies in epidemiology	www.consort-statement.org/index.aspx?o=1065
STROBE statement	Strengthening the reporting of observational studies in epidemiology	www.strobe-statement.org/
TREND statement	Improving the reporting quality of non-randomised evaluations of behavioural and public health interventions	www.trend-statement.org/asp/trend.asp

Table 2-4 **Best study design to answer question**

Type of question	Study design
Therapy	Randomised controlled trial
Prevention	Randomised controlled trial
Aetiology	Randomised controlled trial
Harm	Randomised controlled trial
Prognosis	Cohort study with ≥ 80% follow-up
Diagnosis	Validating cohort study with good reference standards
Differential diagnosis	Prospective cohort study with adequate follow-up
Symptom prevalence study	Prospective cohort study with adequate follow-up

pose challenges in terms of their reliability and relevance to practice. The increasing availability of systematic reviews which combine similar studies from a range of institutions and environments means their relevance to general practice (generalisability) increases.

Key Points

When looking for answers to clinical questions start at the top of the hierarchy and work down:

1. Evidence-based consensus-driven clinical guidelines
2. Cochrane systematic reviews
3. Systematic reviews
4. Studies.

References

Cooper HM. Scientific guidelines for conducting integrative research reviews. Rev Educ Res 1982;52:291–302.

Glass GV. Primary, secondary, and meta-analysis of research. Educ Res 1976;5:3–8.

Higgins JPT, Green S (eds). Cochrane Handbook for Systematic Reviews of Interventions, [updated Sept. 2006]. www.cochrane.org/resources/handbook/hbook.htm (accessed 6 October 2006).

Jackson GB. Methods for integrative reviews. Rev Educ Res 1980;50:438–460.

Khan KS, Riet G, Glanville J, Sowden AJ, Kleijnen J (eds). Undertaking Systematic Reviews of Research on Effectiveness: CRD's Guidance for Carrying Out or Commissioning Reviews. 2nd edn. York: NHS Centre for Reviews and Dissemination, University of York, 2001.

Light RJ, Smith PV. Accumulating evidence: procedures for resolving contradictions among different research studies. Harv Educ Rev 1971;41:429–471.

Mulrow CD. The medical review article: state of the science. Ann Intern Med 1987; 106:485–458.

Olsen O, Middleton P, Ezzo J, Gotzsche PC, Hadhazy V, Herxheimer A et al. Quality of Cochrane reviews: assessment of sample from 1998. Br Med J 2001; 323(7317):829–832.

Oxman AD, Guyatt GH. Guidelines for reading literature reviews. Can Med Assoc J 1988;138:697–703.

Rosenthal R. Combining results of independent studies. Psychol Bull 1978;85: 185–193.

Yusuf S, Simon R, Ellenberg S (eds). Proceedings of methodologic issues in overviews of randomized clinical trials. Stat Med 1987;6:217–409.

Chapter 3
Clinical Scenarios

Aim

This chapter outlines a range of clinical scenarios to enable you to work through the evidence-based process.

Outcome

By outlining how you would respond to these scenarios, you will be able to see how your responses compare with the evidence presented in the subsequent chapters.

Scenario A
A mother with two older children who have had experience of dental decay resulting in fillings and extraction wants to know how the same can be prevented in her newborn (Fig 3-1)?

Scenario B
It is Friday afternoon. An adult patient who is an irregular attender presents with history of a dull throbbing pain in a filled tooth that is tender to percussion. The patient is keen to retain the tooth and is going away for the weekend (Fig 3-2).

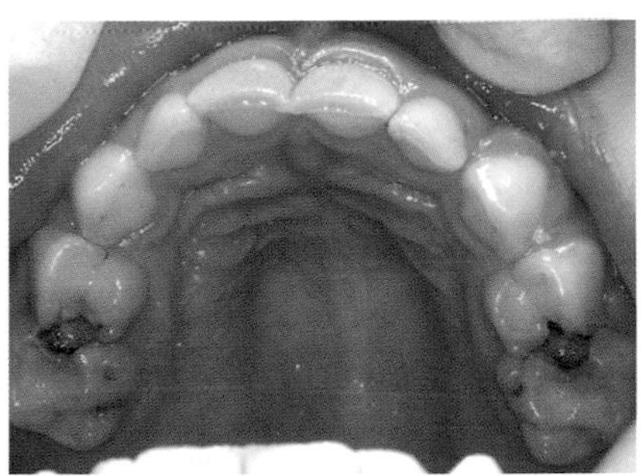

Fig 3-1 Scenario A

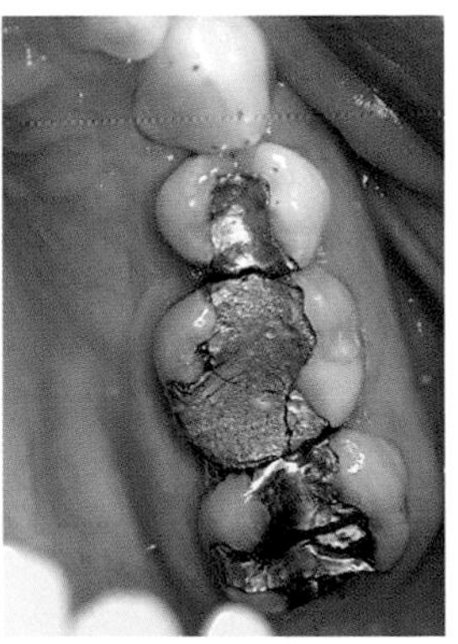

Fig 3-2 Scenario B

Scenario C

The practice has just increased its fees and a regular attender has asked what the benefits are of the scale and polish they receive every time they come for a check-up (Fig 3-3).

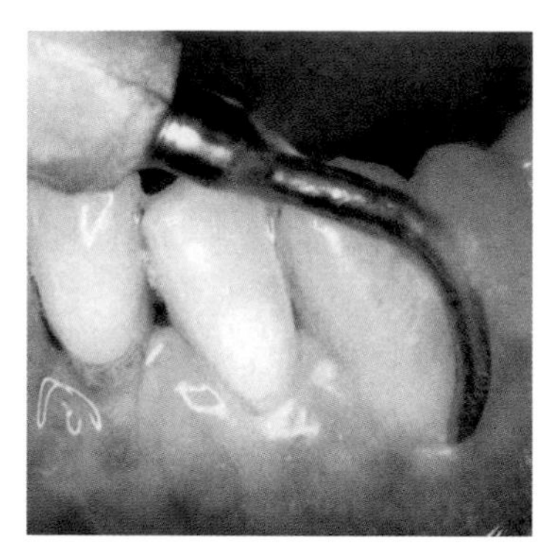

Fig 3-3 Scenario C.

Scenario D

A mother has read on the internet about plastic coatings to protect children's teeth from decay and has asked you whether they work and how long they last (Fig 3-4).

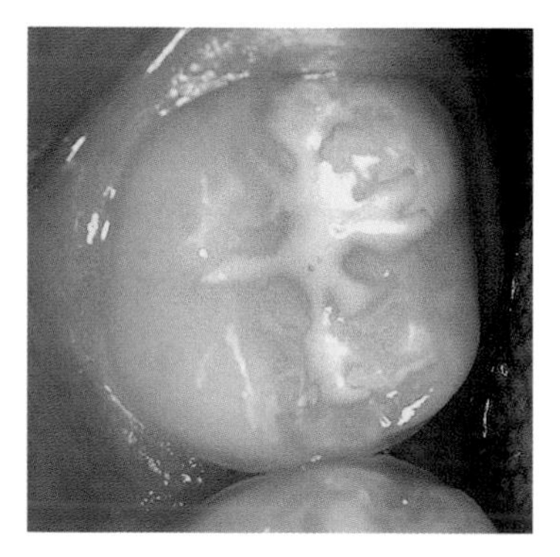

Fig 3-4 Scenario D.

Scenario E

You go to a postgraduate lecture and hear about a new non-invasive technique involving the use of ozone to prevent dental decay. You wonder whether you should invest in the expensive equipment required (Fig 3-5).

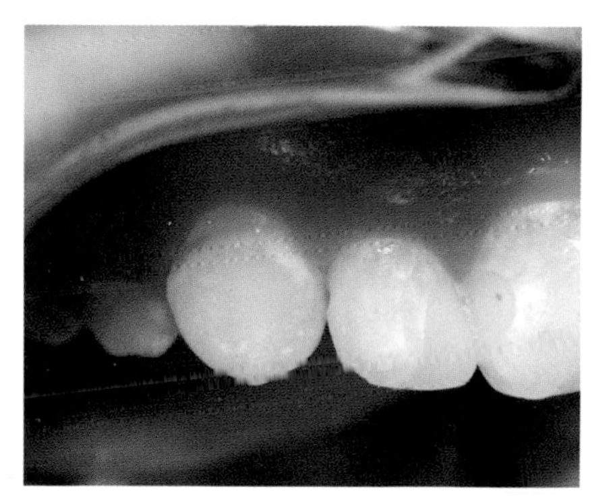

Fig 3-5 Scenario E.

Scenario F

Your practice sells a range of oral health products. A company representative comes to the practice to discuss over lunch their new powered toothbrush. He claims that it is the only one with evidence that it is superior to a manual brush (Fig 3-6).

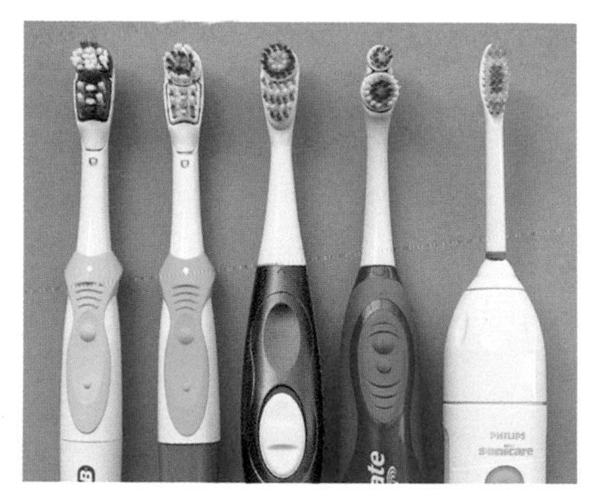

Fig 3-6 Scenario F.

Scenario G

A regularly attending patient is having a routine visit six weeks before her wedding. She is interested in whitening her teeth for the big day but she is concerned about the damage it might cause after reading an article in a women's magazine. Because she is so busy with her wedding plans she is interested in doing it at home rather than arranging another appointment (Fig 3-7).

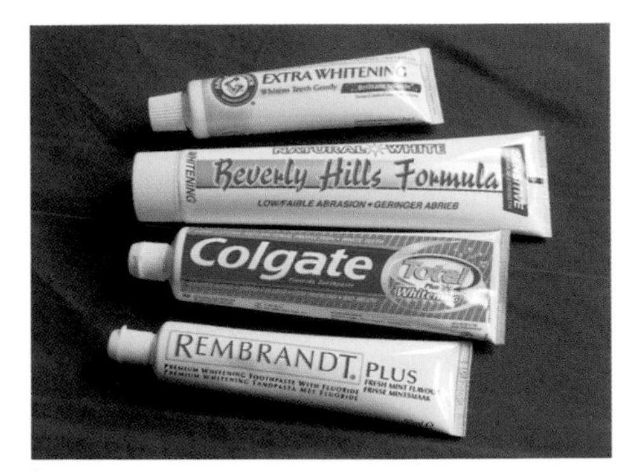

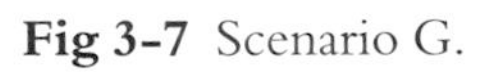
Fig 3-7 Scenario G.

Scenario H

A patient is keen to follow the advice of her health visitor to breastfeed but has heard that it has been linked to early dental decay. What would you advise (Fig 3-8)?

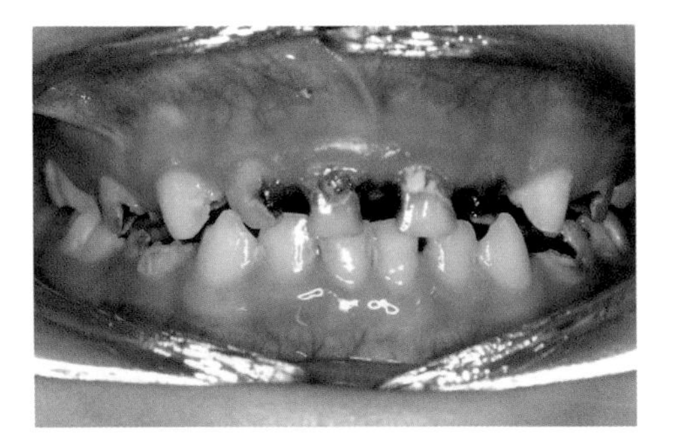

Fig 3-8 Scenario H.

Chapter 4

Evidence-based Guidelines

Aim

The aim of this chapter is to define guidelines, highlight key guideline resources and introduce questions for the appraisal of guidelines.

Outcomes

After completing this chapter readers will be able to define guidelines, be aware of a number of resources to find guidelines and have eight simple questions to help them decide whether to trust a guideline.

Understanding Guidelines

"Guidelines are systematically developed statements which assist in decision making about appropriate health care for specific clinical conditions" (Field and Lohr, 1990).

Well-developed guidelines will have gone through at least the first three stages of the five-stage evidence-based process (Ask, Acquire, Appraise, Apply and Assess). Some will even provide information on when they should be applied and how you assess your outcomes. In this chapter we take you through where to look for them and how to decide if they can be trusted.

Let us consider the first two scenarios outlined in Chapter 3, and apply the evidence-based method.

Scenario A
A mother with two older children who have had experience of dental decay resulting in fillings and extraction wants to know how the same can be prevented in her newborn (Fig 4-1)?

Scenario B
It is Friday afternoon. An adult patient who is an irregular attender presents with history of a dull throbbing pain in a filled tooth that is tender to

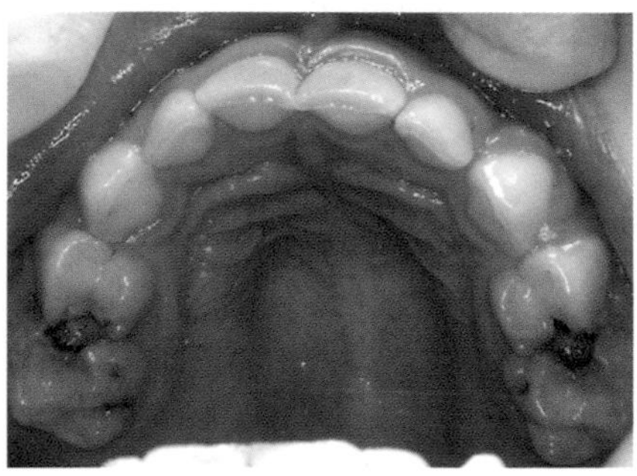

Fig 4-1 Scenario A, prevention of decay.

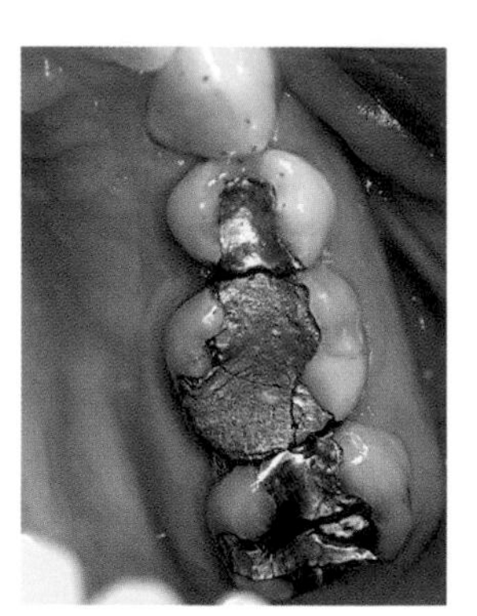

Fig 4-2 Scenario B, pain in a filled tooth.

percussion. The patient is keen to retain the tooth and is going away for the weekend (Fig 4-2).

First we need to confirm what the question is – the ASK stage.

While the question in scenario A may seem obvious to the experienced practitioner, it may not necessarily be the question to which the patient actually needs an answer. For example, in this case the questions the mother might want answered are:

- When should I start brushing my child's teeth?
- When should children start brushing their own teeth?
- Should I use fluoridated toothpaste?
- How much toothpaste should I use?
- Should I use fluoride tablets?
- What about fluorosis?
- Can my child have sweets?
- What foods and drinks should I avoid giving my child?
- Is there anything the dentist can do to help?
- What about my older children?

PICO (PECO)

A useful method of clarifying the question is to use the PICO format (Richardson et al., 1995). PICO is a useful acronym that describes the elements of a well-formed clinical question about therapy. The letters stand for:

Population, patient or problem
Intervention or treatment, or **E**xposure or potential risk factor
Comparison
Outcome

Population is really a general description of the group to which your patient belongs, and may include age, gender, race, ethnicity and stage of disease. The description should be specific enough to be helpful, but not overly specific. You are unlikely to find studies of "Asian 63-year-old women" (too specific); describing the population as "post-menopausal women" is much more likely to be helpful. When reading or searching for clinical evidence, this term helps you determine whether you can apply the evidence you find to the group of patients you deal with on a regular basis.

Intervention/exposure is a description of the test or treatment (or exposure to a potential risk factor) that you are considering. This is the most useful term to use when searching databases or websites for the best available evidence.

Comparison is the alternative intervention or exposure. It may be the current gold standard treatment, a placebo or watchful waiting (i.e. monitoring, no treatment). Not all questions need a comparison but, in terms of treatment, the only way we can be certain that a new method or material is better than what we are currently using (or than nothing at all) is to use a comparison group.

Outcome refers to what we are expecting to find as a result of the treatment or exposure. Are you looking to see an improvement in the quality of life, a reduction in dental caries, an association between a potential cause and effect, or whether a new diagnostic test adds to the confidence of your diagnosis?

Most research studies deal with clinical outcomes like millimetres of probing depth or bond strength, but the outcome should be something that not only matters to you but matters to the patient too. (Do patients really care if you can reduce their probing pocket depths by 0.68 mm? Or are they more interested in how long they can keep their teeth?)

Defining the outcome is not necessarily helpful in searching for the answers, but once you find some studies that look at this question, you can eliminate (not have to read!) the ones that don't deal with the outcome of interest.

Scenario A

A mother with two older children who have had experience of dental decay resulting in fillings and extraction wants to know how the same can be prevented in her newborn.

Population	Intervention	Comparison	Outcomes
Pre-school children	Caries prevention methods • topical fluorides • toothpaste • fluoridation • dietary advice	Caries prevention methods • topical fluorides • toothpaste • fluoridation • dietary advice	Reduction in caries Quality of life measures

Applying the PICO format as shown in the grid to Scenario A gives the PICO question: *In pre-school children what is the best method for preventing caries?* Alternatively: *How can you prevent caries in the pre-school child?*

As dental healthcare professionals, we know that there are several methods and approaches to prevent caries, so this is a good reason to start our search for evidence with an evidence-based guideline.

The best place to search for guidelines is the National Guideline Clearinghouse™ (NGC). This is a fairly comprehensive database of evidence-based clinical practice guidelines and related documents. The NGC is an initiative of the Agency for Healthcare Research and Quality (AHRQ), US Department of Health and Human Services. The NGC can be found at www.guidelines.gov.

The NGC has a simple search function on the home page (Fig 4-3). Searching using the term "dental caries" indicates 39 references, the first two of which are:

- *Prevention of dental caries in preschool children: recommendations and rationale. United States Preventive Services Task Force – Independent Expert Panel. 1989 (revised 2004 Apr 8). 9 pages. NGC:003184.*
- *Prevention and management of dental decay in the pre-school child. A national clinical guideline. Scottish Intercollegiate Guidelines Network – National Government Agency [Non-U.S.]. 2005 Nov. 41 pages. NGC:004703.*

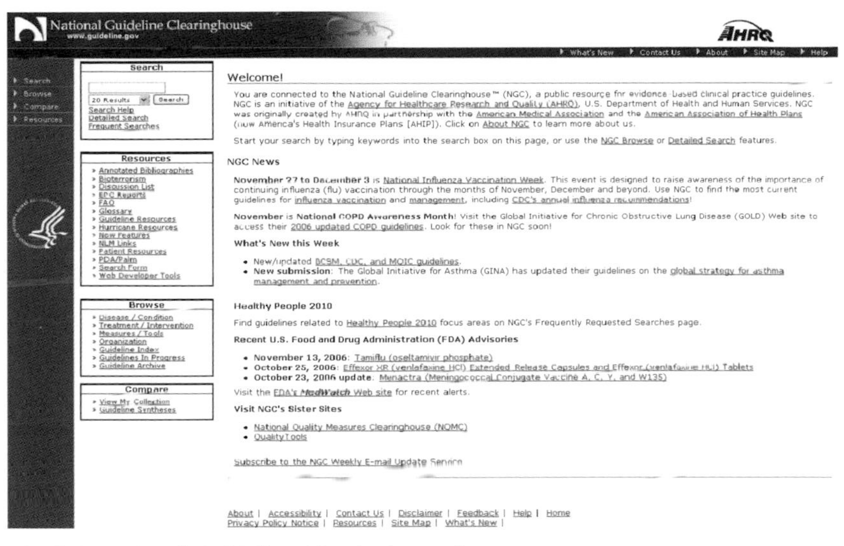

Fig 4-3 National Guideline Clearinghouse home page.

Both seem relevant to the question but the second guideline was published in 2005 and therefore likely to contain the most recent evidence. Clicking the reference title takes you to a detailed summary of the main recommendations. This page also has links to the Scottish Intercollegiate Guidelines Network (SIGN) website (www.sign.ac.uk) who are the developers of this guideline.

On this website a quick reference guide and the full guideline are available for download in portable document format (PDF). Having identified an evidence-based clinical guideline to complete the ACQUIRE stage we must now decide if it can be trusted – the APPRAISE stage.

Appraisal is an extremely important step. Even though a guideline claims to be evidence-based it doesn't mean the evidence is very strong, or that the guideline development process was rigorous. Knowing the key factors to look for in a guideline will allow you more confidence that the guideline is useful. A detailed tool for appraising guidelines can be obtained from the AGREE (Appraisal of Guidelines Research and Evaluation) website (www.agreecollaboration.org). A rapid assessment can, however, be made using the questions in Table 4-1.

Table 4-1 **Can I trust this guideline?**

Answer the eight questions; yes, no, not sure. The more green boxes marked the more you can trust the guideline.			
	Yes	**No**	**Not sure**
1. Is the guideline easy to read and easy to follow?			
2. Does it address a clearly defined clinical topic?			
3. Did the authors follow a documented evidence-based system for producing the guideline?			
4. Or did the authors just add references to their own opinions?			
5. Was the evidence found via a systematic and documented search of all relevant literature?			
6. Has the evidence been appraised and graded for quality?			
7. Is the evidence regularly and systematically updated?			
8. Can you link directly to the evidence – all the references – that underpin each major treatment option?			

When you are happy you can trust the guideline you have then reached the APPLY stage of the evidence-based method.

The quick reference guide is an easy-to-read two-page document and could easily be used at the chair-side with the parent to discuss the right options to be used in her particular circumstances. This discussion phase where the evidence, clinical experience and patients' values are considered is a key feature of the evidence-based approach and marks it out from a simple matter of blindly following the evidence.

The final step in the evidence-based method closes the loop (the ASSESSMENT stage). This could be an assessment of how you conducted the process, with any learning points for yourself, what the outcomes were for the patient, or the impact adopting the guideline had on the practice. If the guideline is valid you might even follow some of the suggestions for audit in the main document.

Scenario B

It is Friday afternoon. An adult patient who is an irregular attender presents with a history of dull throbbing pain in a filled tooth that is tender to percussion. The patient is keen to retain the tooth and is going away for the weekend.

Population	Intervention	Comparison	Outcomes
Adults with acute apical periodontitis (AAP)	*Systemic* and *local* pharmacotherapeutics including: • *Systemic* (antibiotics, corticosteroids, NSAIDS/analgesics) and • *Local* (irrigants, intracanal medicaments) therapy pulpectomy, open or closed bony trephina-tion extraction, occlusal adjustment and "watchful wait-ing" (no treatment)	*Systemic* and *local* pharmacotherapeutics including: • *Systemic* (antibiotics, corticosteroids, NSAIDS/analgesics) and • *Local* (irrigants, intracanal medicaments) therapy pulpectomy, open or closed bony trepina-tion extraction, occlusal adjustment and "watchful wait-ing" (no treatment)	Reduction in pain Tooth retained/lost

This case is one that will be familiar to many; examination shows a defective restoration with secondary caries in a lower first permanent molar. A radiograph shows the carious lesion and probably pulpal exposure but no periapical radiolucency or periodontal widening. A range of potential treatments is available, but which one has the best supporting evidence?

This is an area where a known clinical guideline exists, yet it does not appear on the NGC's extensive website. A useful alternative site to the NGC website for searching for high-quality dental guidelines is Oral Health Specialist Library (www.library.nhs.uk/oralhealth) (Fig 4-4).

Searching for "apical periodontitis" in the search box identifies one guideline and clicking on the "view details" links takes you to a summary of the recommendations (Box 4-1).

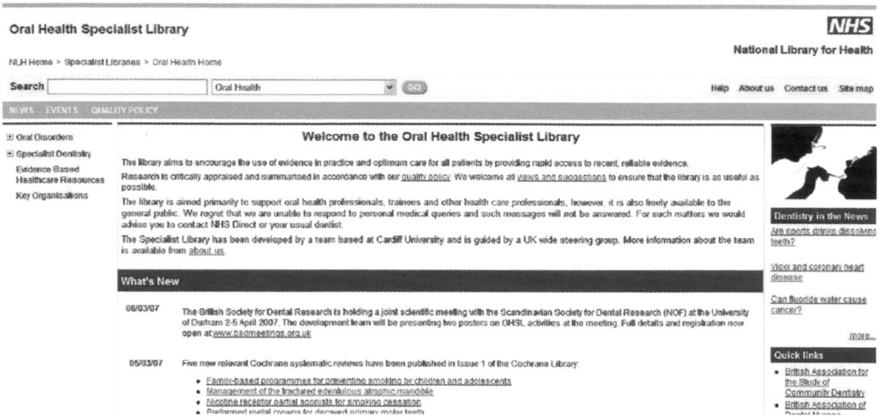

Fig 4-4 Oral Health Specialist Library.

Box 4-1 **Emergency management of acute apical periodontitis in adults**

Recommendations

- Non-surgical endodontic therapy (root canal) should be started on the affected tooth as soon as possible.
- Patients should be given the appropriate dose of analgesics (NSAIDs if not contraindicated) preoperatively, or immediately post-operatively. This should be continued as needed to control pain.
- In the event that endodontic therapy cannot be started immediately, appropriate analgesics should be prescribed.
- For some patients, extraction may be an alternative to endodontic therapy.
- If the tooth is in hyper-occlusion, the occlusion should be relieved if possible.
- Non-surgical endodontic therapy (root canal) should be started on the affected tooth as soon as possible.
- Antibiotic therapy is not indicated for this condition.
- Bony trephination is not indicated for this condition.

This guideline was developed by the Canadian Collaboration on Clinical Practice Guidelines in Dentistry (CCCD) which is sadly no longer operating. If, instead of clicking the view details link, the evidence link is clicked, this will take the viewer to two systematic reviews with a link to the original systematic review (Sutherland and Matthews, 2003) which was carried out to inform the development of the guideline.

The Oral Health Specialist Library has a very clear quality process which can be seen by clicking the appropriate link. Because of this the practitioner can use the guideline. However, an appraisal does need to be made about whether it is appropriate to use the guidance with this patient.

As with the SIGN caries guideline, in terms of the assessment phase of the evidence-based method you could consider auditing how many scripts for analgesia rather than antibiotics you write as a result of reading this guideline.

Key Points

- The number of good-quality guidelines in dentistry are increasing and they should be the first port of call for the busy practitioner.
- A simple eight-question test can help you decide whether to trust the guideline.
- Many of the guidelines are freely available on the internet. The Centre for Evidence-based Dentistry provides links to them at: www.cebd.org/?o=1067
- Guidelines must be applied taking into account your patient's values and preferences, as well as his or her medical and dental history.

References

Field MJ, Lohr KN (eds). Clinical Practice Guidelines: Directions for a New Program. Institute of Medicine, Washington, DC: National Academy Press, 1990.

Richardson W, Wilson M, Nishikawa J, Hayward RS. The well-built clinical question: a key to evidence-based decisions [editorial]. ACP J Club 1995;123:A12–13.

Sutherland S, Matthews DC. Emergency management of acute apical periodontitis in the permanent dentition: a systematic review of the literature. J Can Dent Assoc 2003;69:160.

Additional Reading

GRADE Working Group. Grading quality of evidence and strength of recommendations. Br Med J 2004; 328(7454):1490.

GRADE Working Group. Systems for grading the quality of evidence and the strength of recommendations I: critical appraisal of existing approaches. The GRADE Working Group. BMC Health Serv Res 2004;4(1):38.

GRADE Working Group. Systems for grading the quality of evidence and the strength of recommendations II: pilot study of a new system. BMC Health Serv Res 2005;5(1):25.

Sutherland SE, Matthews DC, Fendrich P. Clinical practice guidelines in dentistry: Part I. Navigating new waters. J Can Dent Assoc 2001;67(7):379–383.

Sutherland SE, Matthews DC. Conducting systematic reviews and creating clinical practice guidelines in dentistry: lessons learned. J Am Dent Assoc 2004;135(6): 747–753.

Chapter 5

Cochrane Reviews

Aim

The aim of this chapter is to show the reader how to find and appraise Cochrane systematic reviews using the Cochrane Library and introduce them to the Cochrane Collaboration and Cochrane Oral Health Group.

Outcomes

After completing this chapter readers should be aware of the Cochrane Collaboration, Library and Oral Health Group and have ten questions to help them appraise a systematic review.

Finding and Assessing Cochrane Systematic Reviews

Guidelines are unlikely to be available for every clinical situation in dentistry. Systematic reviews which summarise the available evidence are more widely available and cover a wide range of topics. Systematic reviews prepared by the Cochrane Collaboration are the highest quality systematic reviews available. Here we show you where to look for them and how to assess them.

Scenario C
The practice has just increased its fees and a regular attender has asked what the benefits are of the scale and polish they receive every time they come for a check-up.

Scenario D
A mother has read on the internet about plastic coatings to protect children's teeth from decay and has asked you whether they work and how long they last.

Scenario E
You go to a postgraduate lecture and hear about a new non-invasive technique involving the use of ozone to prevent dental decay. You wonder whether you should invest in the expensive equipment required.

Scenario F

Your practice sells a range of oral health products. A company rep comes to the practice to discuss over lunch their new powered toothbrush. He claims that it is the only one with evidence that it is superior to a manual brush.

If you didn't write down your answers to scenarios C–D before you read the chapter then consider them now. As before, the first stage is the ASK.

Scenario C

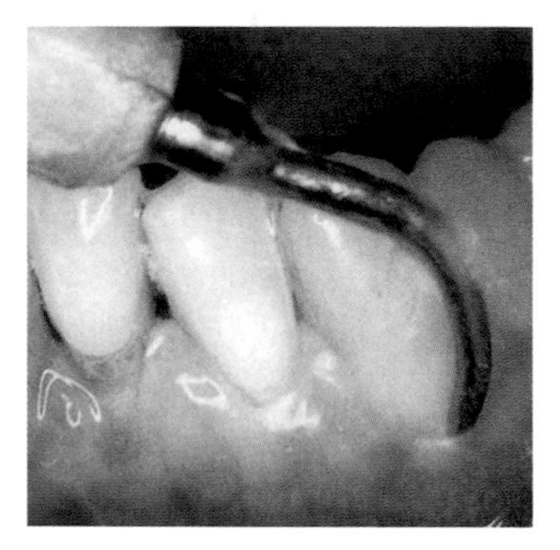

Fig 5-1 Scenario C, scale and polish.

The practice has just increased its fees and a regular attender has asked what the benefits are of the scale and polish he receives every time he comes for a check-up.

Population	Intervention	Comparison	Outcomes
Adults (regular attenders)	Scale and polish	No scale and polish	Improved gingival health Reduction in periodontal disease BOP; pocket depth; attachment loss Quality of life measures

In this case you may also like to consider disadvantages as some patients don't like having scale and polish, so you should also consider pain and post-operative discomfort!

ACQUIRE

Scale and polish is a specific treatment or intervention – for specific interventions or treatments the Cochrane Library (see page 115) is a good place to start (Fig 5-2).

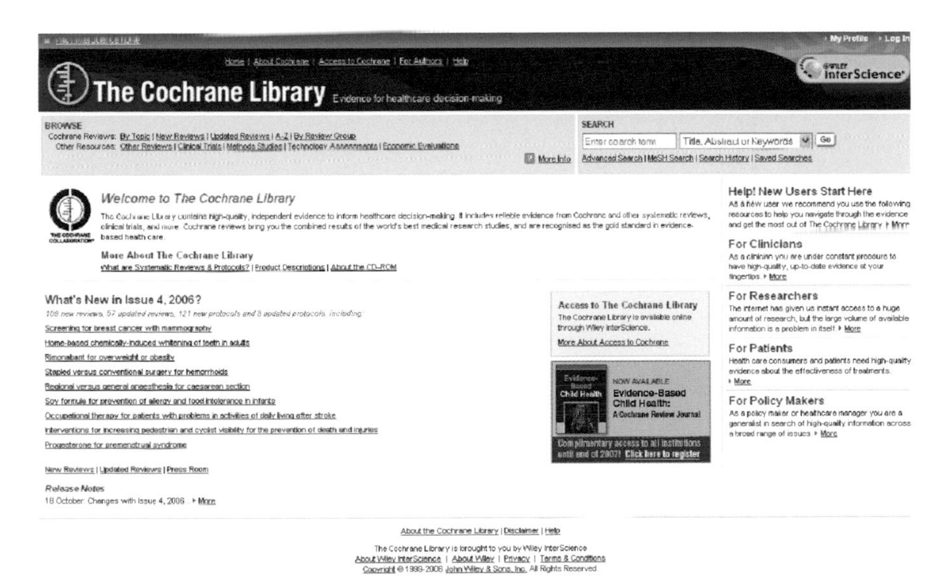

Fig 5-2 The Cochrane Library homepage.

Searching the Cochrane Library is similar to searching most internet sites. The home page has a simple search box, but a more advanced searching facility is available.

Putting the term "scale and polish" in the simple search box and pressing search will bring up only two references as seen in Fig 5-3. Scale and polish is such a specifically dental term that using the simple search strategy is sufficient.

A small [redacted image] image shows that a review is available and when the hypertext word *record* is clicked on, the review abstract is shown. Scrolling down to the bottom of the abstract will enable you to read the authors' conclusions and, at the end, a plain language summary (see Box 5-1).

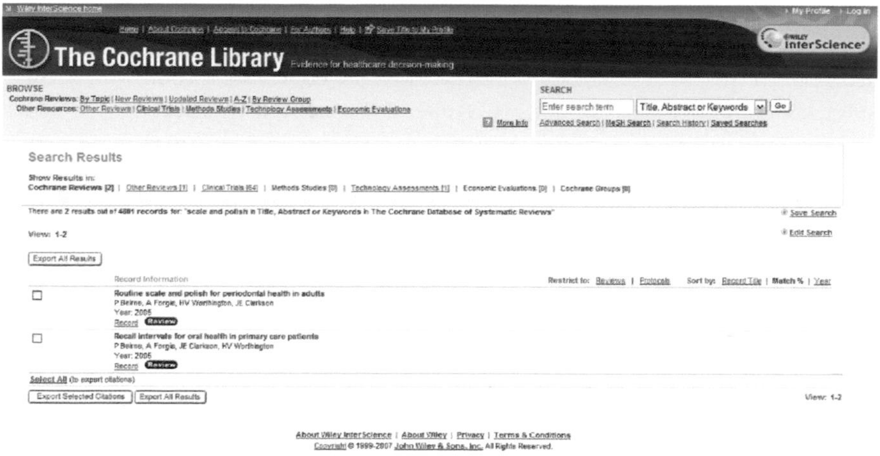

Fig 5-3 The Cochrane Library – showing the scale and polish search.

Box 5-1 **Routine scale and polish for periodontal health in adults**

Authors' conclusions

The research evidence is of insufficient quality to reach any conclusions regarding the beneficial and adverse effects of routine scaling and polishing for periodontal health and regarding the effects of providing this intervention at different time intervals. High-quality clinical trials are required to address the basic questions posed in this review.

Plain language summary

The effects on periodontal health of a routine scale and polish and of providing this intervention at different time intervals are unclear.

Many dentists and hygienists regularly provide scaling and polishing for patients, even if those patients are considered to be at low risk of developing periodontal (gum) disease. The trials included in this review were judged to be of poor quality. The research evidence was of insufficient quality to reach any conclusions regarding the beneficial and adverse effects of routine scaling and polishing for periodontal health and regarding the effects of providing this intervention at different time intervals.

Beirne P, Forgie A, Worthington HV, Clarkson JE. Routine scale and polish for periodontal health in adults. Cochrane Database of Systematic Reviews 2005, Issue 1. Art. No.: CD004625. DOI: 10.1002/14651858.CD004625.pub2.

Note: Within the confines of this Cochrane review a "routine scale and polish" is defined as scaling and/or polishing of the crown and root surfaces of teeth to remove local irritational factors (plaque, calculus, debris and staining), that does not involve periodontal surgery or any form of adjunctive periodontal therapy such as the use of chemotherapeutic agents or root planing.

Once you have identified a review to answer your question it would normally need to be appraised before you apply it to your patients. Cochrane reviews are of high quality, being conducted according to strict protocols with high standards of peer review and can therefore be accepted as best evidence. The abstracts of Cochrane reviews provide much more information than a normal abstract so are usually sufficiently detailed to give you a rapid answer to your clinical problem. In the UK and several other countries the whole review can be read online or downloaded in PDF format (access to the Cochrane Library varies from country to country – see (www3.interscience.wiley.com/cgi-bin/mrwhome/106568753/AccessCochraneLibrary.html) for details.

APPRAISE

While Cochrane reviews can be accepted as best evidence it is useful to consider how you would appraise a review. A number of different appraisal tools are available on the internet. One such set are those developed by CASP, the Critical Appraisal Skills Programme (www.phru.nhs.uk/Pages/PHD/resources.htm), which has been helping to develop an evidence-based approach in health and social care, working with local, national and international groups.

For reviews CASP has developed 10 questions (Fig 5-4) adapted from a paper by Oxman et al. (1994). The questions address three broad issues:

- Is the study valid?
- What are the results?
- Will the results help locally?

Questions 1 and 2 are designed to be screening questions and if you answer no to both of these it is unlikely to be worth continuing. Questions 3, 4 and 5 address the validity of the study. Questions 6 and 7 identify the results of the study, while the last three questions are important to help you decide whether you can and should use the information to amend your practice in light of the evidence presented.

APPLY

From the Cochrane review it is evident that the quality of evidence relating to the positive and negative effects of routine scaling and polishing is limited. Therefore, a discussion needs to take place between the dentist and the patient (a patient in the UK would be able to access the Cochrane Library and obtain exactly the same information as the dentist assuming that they

		Yes	No	Can't tell
1.	Did the review ask a clearly-focused question?	☐	☐	☐
2.	Did the review include the right type of study?	☐	☐	☐
3.	Did the reviewers try to identify all relevant studies?	☐	☐	☐
4.	Did the reviewers assess the quality of the included studies?	☐	☐	☐
5.	If the results of the studies have been combined, was it reasonable to do so?	☐	☐	☐
6.	How are the results presented and what is the main result?	----------------		
7.	How precise are these results?	----------------		
8.	Can the results be applied to the local population?	☐	☐	☐
9.	Were all important outcomes considered?	☐	☐	☐
10.	Should policy or practice change as a result of the evidence contained in this review?	☐	☐	☐

Fig 5-4 CASP 10 questions to help you make sense of reviews.

have access to the internet), in order to agree whether (based on the evidence, clinical circumstances and patient's wishes) a scale and polish is provided for that patient.

ASSESS

The impact of applying this evidence can be assessed on either an individual patient basis or potentially on your practice.

Scenario D

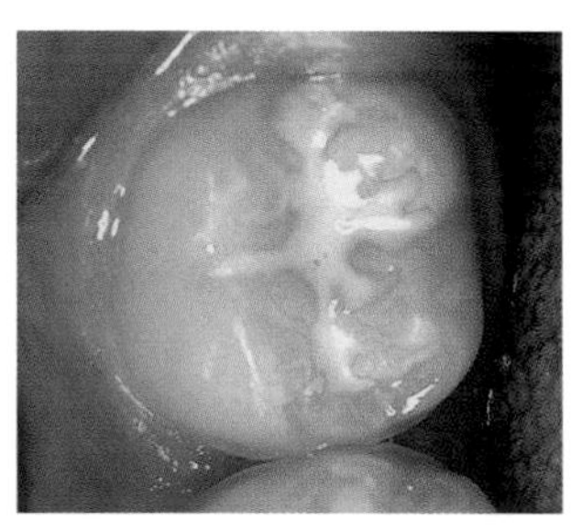

Fig 5-5 Scenario D, fissure sealants.

A mother has read on the internet about the plastic coatings to protect children's teeth from decay and has asked you whether they work and how long they last.

Population	Intervention	Comparison	Outcomes
Children	Fissure sealants	No treatment Other preventive treatments	Reduced decay Sealant retention

ASK

The questions here can be written as:

- Do fissure sealants reduce decay in occlusal surfaces?
- How long are dental sealants retained?
- Are fissure sealants more effective than other preventive treatments?

ACQUIRE

A simple search, using the term *fissure sealants*, on the Cochrane Library shows two completed reviews.

Looking at the plain language summaries of both reviews (Boxes 5-2 and 5-3), the first review clearly shows that sealing teeth between the ages of 5–10 years showed a reduction in decay in the occlusal surfaces of permanent teeth of over 50%.

The second review suggests that sealants are better than fluoride varnish applications but the number of available studies are low.

Box 5-2 **Pit and fissure sealants for preventing dental decay in the permanent teeth of children and adolescents**

Plain language summary

The review shows that after 4.5 years the sealed permanent molar teeth of children aged 5 to 10 had a reduction of decay in over 50% of biting surfaces compared to teeth without sealants.

Ahovuo-Saloranta A, Hiiri A, Nordblad A, Worthington H, Mäkelä M. Pit and fissure sealants for preventing dental decay in the permanent teeth of children and adolescents. *Cochrane Database of Systematic Reviews* 2004, Issue 3. Art. No.: CD001830. DOI: 10.1002/14651858.CD001830.pub2.

Box 5-3 **Pit and fissure sealants versus fluoride varnishes for preventing dental decay in children and adolescents**

Plain language summary

Dental sealants reduce more tooth decay in the grooves of back teeth in children than fluoride varnish application but the number of studies supporting this evidence are very low.

Sealants are coatings applied by the dentist or by another person in dental care on the grooves of back teeth. These coatings are intended to prevent decay in the grooves of back teeth.

Fluoride varnishes are sticky pastes that are professionally applied on teeth at a frequency of two to four times a year. The review found that dental sealants reduce more tooth decay in grooves of permanent teeth than fluoride varnishes. However, more high-quality research is needed to clarify how big the difference is between the effectiveness of pit and fissure sealants and fluoride varnishes.

Hiiri A, Ahovuo-Saloranta A, Nordblad A, Mäkelä M. Pit and fissure sealants versus fluoride varnishes for preventing dental decay in children and adolescents. *Cochrane Database of Systematic Reviews* 2006, Issue 4. Art. No.: CD003067. DOI: 10.1002/14651858.CD003067.pub2.

APPRAISE and APPLY

Both of these Cochrane reviews indicate that fissure sealants are effective at reducing caries and appraisal of the review can be undertaken using the 10 questions noted previously. (Other Cochrane reviews indicate that fluoride varnish is very effective at reducing caries (Marinho et al., 2002) and that other preventive measures are additive so can be combined (Marinho et al., 2004)).

Your decision to use sealants should be based on this evidence and the clinical situation. Well-quoted guidance on sealant placement is available from the British Society of Paediatric Dentistry (Nunn et al., 2000). Interested readers may wish to appraise the BSPD guideline using the tool in Chapter 4.

ASSESS

As previously, assessing whether to use this evidence-based practice could be decided by auditing the proportion of children in your practice requiring sealants who had had them placed. The BSPD guidelines could be a useful starting-point although you could develop some for your own practice. While one of the reviews reports data at 4.5 years, this is limited information about how long sealants last or their reapplication. Therefore sealant retention is another potential audit that could be conducted within the practice.

Scenario E

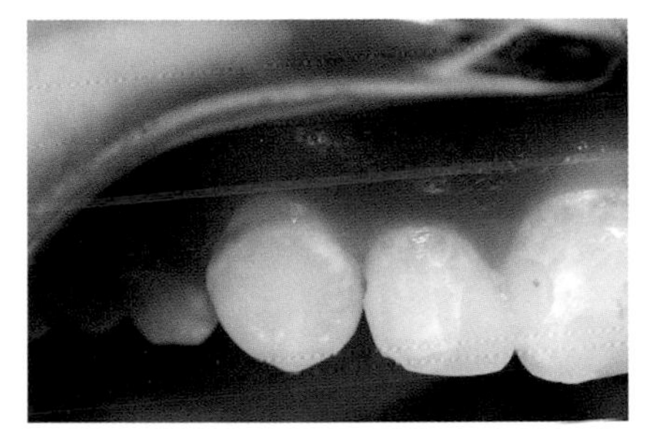

Fig 5-6 Scenario E, ozone to prevent decay.

You go to a postgraduate lecture and hear about a new non-invasive technique involving the use of ozone to prevent dental decay. You wonder whether you should invest in the expensive equipment required.

Population	Intervention	Comparison	Outcomes
People at risk of dental decay	Ozone therapy	Other preventive treatments	Arrest decay Prevent decay

ASK

The question can be broken down into various elements as shown or summarised as:

- Does ozone therapy arrest or prevent dental decay?

ACQUIRE

Again a simple search of the Cochrane Library using the term *ozone* identified one review which was completed in 2004 (Box 5-4).

APPRAISE and APPLY

Based on this review, it would seem prudent to wait for the additional research to be completed before considering the purchase of additional equipment.

This view is supported by a heath technology appraisal conducted by the NHS National Institute for Health and Clinical Excellence (NICE) and published in 2005. The summary is shown below (Box 5-5) but the full details can be found at www.nice.org.uk/page.aspx?o=TA92. NICE plans to review this in 2008.

Box 5-4 **Ozone therapy for the treatment of dental caries**

> **Plain language summary**
>
> It has been suggested that treatment of a decayed tooth with ozone will stop or reverse the decay process. This review of trials found no sound evidence that ozone is capable of reversing or stopping the progression of tooth decay. High-quality research is needed to show whether or not it works. Ozone should not be considered an alternative to current treatment methods in dental practices.
>
> Rickard GD, Richardson R, Johnson T, McColl D, Hooper L. Ozone therapy for the treatment of dental caries. *Cochrane Database of Systematic Reviews* 2004, Issue 3. Art. No.: CD004153. DOI: 10.1002/14651858.CD004153.pub2.

Box 5-5 **Ozone therapy for the treatment of dental caries**

> **Summary**
>
> NICE declares that HealOzone is not recommended as a treatment for specific types of tooth decay, unless it is being used in a clinical trial.
>
> The reason for this was that there was not enough reliable evidence that HealOzone is more effective than existing treatments for decay of the biting surfaces and roots of the teeth.14651858.CD004153.pub2.

Scenario F

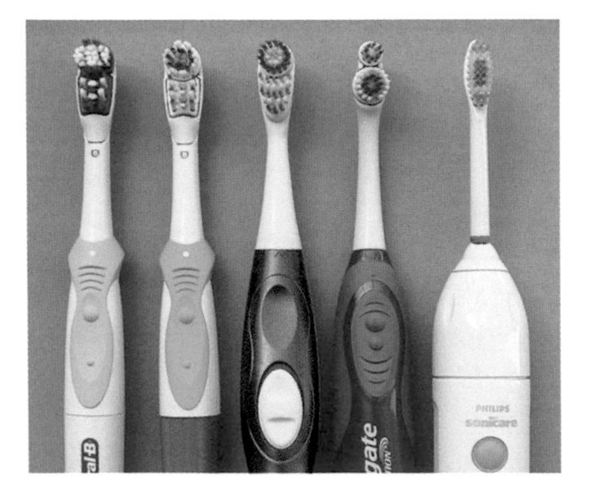

Fig 5-7 Scenario F, powered toothbrushes.

Your practice sells a range of oral health products. A company representative comes to the practice to discuss their new powered toothbrush over lunch. He claims that it is the only one with evidence that it is superior to a manual brush.

Population	Intervention	Comparison	Outcomes
Dentate patients	Powered toothbrush	Manual toothbrush	Improved oral health, gingivitis (periodontal disease) and caries

ASK

While it may be tempting to focus on the particular brand name for the brush it would be wiser to start looking a little wider to see if powered toothbrushes are better than manual brushes before looking at a specific manufacturer's brush. It is likely that the number of studies on a particular brand will be small and the majority will have been supported by that manufacturer.

The question can be broken down into its constituent parts as shown below and summarised as:

- Will the use of a powered toothbrush compared to a manual toothbrush result in improved oral health (reduction in plaque and gingivitis)?

ACQUIRE

A simple search on the Cochrane Library using the term *powered toothbrush* yields three references, two reviews and one protocol. One review is directly relevant to the question being asked. The main results, authors' conclusions and plain language summary are shown in Box 5-6.

APPRAISE and APPLY

As before, the additional information provided by Cochrane abstracts and the quality of the development and peer review process within the Cochrane Collaboration means that there are unlikely to be significant methodological issues. It is therefore reasonable to concentrate on the results.

What the review finds is that: "*powered toothbrushes whose action is rotation oscillational reduce plaque and gingivitis by 11% and 6% respectively in the short term and gingivitis by 17% at greater than 3 months*".

Box 5-6 **Manual versus powered toothbrushing for oral health**

Main results

Forty-two trials, involving 3855 participants, provided data. Brushes with a rotation oscillation action removed plaque and reduced gingivitis more effectively than manual brushes in the short term and reduced gingivitis scores in studies over three months.

For plaque at one to three months the SMD was –0.43 (95% CI: –0.72 to –0.14); for gingivitis SMD was –0.62 (95% CI: –0.90 to –0.34) representing an 11% difference on the Quigley Hein plaque index and a 6% reduction on the Löe and Silness gingival index. At over three months the SMD for plaque was –1.29 (95% CI: –2.67 to 0.08) and for gingivitis was –0.51 (–0.76 to –0.25) representing a 17% reduction on the Ainamo Bay bleeding on probing index.

There was heterogeneity between the trials for the short-term follow-up. Sensitivity analyses revealed the results to be robust when selecting trials of high quality. There was no evidence of any publication bias.

Authors' conclusions

Powered toothbrushes with a rotation oscillation action reduce plaque and gingivitis more than manual toothbrushing. Observation of methodological guidelines and greater standardisation of design would benefit both future trials and meta-analyses.

Plain language summary

When compared to manual toothbrushes, powered toothbrushes with a rotation oscillation action provide protection against gum inflammation in the long and short term and better plaque removal in the short term. Removing dental plaque by toothbrushing helps prevent gum inflammation (gingivitis). Toothbrushing with a fluoride toothpaste prevents tooth decay. Powered toothbrushes simulate manual toothbrushing in different ways (such as moving side to side or circular motions).

The review of trials found that only rotation oscillation (where brush heads rotate in one direction and then the other) is better than manual toothbrushes at removing plaque and reducing gum inflammation, and is no more likely to cause injuries to gums. Long-term benefits of this for dental health are unclear.

Robinson PG, Deacon SA, Deery C, Heanue M, Walmsley AD, Worthington HV, Glenny AM, Shaw WC. Manual versus powered toothbrushing for oral health. *Cochrane Database of Systematic Reviews* 2005, Issue 2. Art. No.: CD002281. DOI: 10.1002/14651858.CD002281.pub2.

In answer to our question then: if the brush being offered by the sales representative is of the rotational oscillational type, there is good evidence that it will reduce plaque and gingivitis more than using a manual brush. However, we do not know how important this is clinically as the follow-up period is only three months, which is too short term to demonstrate any reduction in destructive periodontal disease.

The review also suggests that it is this particular type of brush (rotational oscillational) rather than a particular brand. Therefore even if this sales representative's brush is of this type he is incorrect to claim that his brush is the only one with evidence to show its superiority over manual brushes.

The Cochrane Collaboration

The Cochrane Collaboration (www.cochrane.org) is an international, non-profit, independent organisation, established in 1993, and named after the epidemiologist, Archie Cochrane (1909–1988). The Collaboration aims to provide up-to-date, accurate information about the effects of healthcare interventions.

The Cochrane Collaboration prepares Cochrane reviews and aims to update them regularly with the latest scientific evidence. Members of the organisation (mostly volunteers) work together to provide evidence to help people make decisions about healthcare.

The major product of the Collaboration is the *Cochrane Database of Systematic Reviews* which is published quarterly as part of The Cochrane Library. With 50 sub-groups, the Collaboration publishes reviews on all aspects of healthcare including oral health.

Cochrane Oral Health Group

The Cochrane Oral Health Group (COHG) registered with The Cochrane Collaboration in June 1994. The editorial base was initially set up in the USA under the coordinating editorship of Alexia Antczak Bouckoms. In August 1996 the editorial base was transferred to the UK within Manchester University's School of Dentistry, with Helen Worthington and Bill Shaw as coordinating editors.

The COHG produces systematic reviews which primarily include all randomised controlled trials (RCTs) of oral health. COHG protocols (details of planned reviews) and reviews are published on The Cochrane Library along with a trials register which is submitted every quarter for publication in the Cochrane Central Register of Controlled Trials which is also held on The Cochrane Library. More details about the work and activities of the COHG can be found on its website (www.ohg.cochrane.org).

Key Points

- Cochrane reviews are a high-quality source of evidence and increasing numbers are available of relevance to dentistry.
- The quality of the Cochrane process and the ready availability of the abstracts can provide rapid answers to clinical problems.
- Cochrane reviews have useful short plain language summaries.

References

Marinho VCC, Higgins JPT, Logan S, Sheiham A. Fluoride varnishes for preventing dental caries in children and adolescents. Cochrane Database of Systematic Reviews 2002, Issue 1. Art. No.: CD002279. DOI: 10.1002/14651858.CD002279.

Marinho VCC, Higgins JPT, Sheiham A, Logan S. Combinations of topical fluoride (toothpastes, mouthrinses, gels, varnishes) versus single topical fluoride for preventing dental caries in children and adolescents. Cochrane Database of Systematic Reviews 2004, Issue 1. Art. No.: CD002781. DOI: 10.1002/ 14651858.CD002781.pub2.

Nunn JH, Murray JJ, Smallridge J. The British Society of Paediatric Dentistry: a policy document on fissure sealants in paediatric dentistry. Int J Paed Dent 2000;10:174–177 (available at www.bspd.co.uk/ publications.html).

Oxman AD, Cook DJ, Guyatt GH. Users' guides to the medical literature. VI. How to use an overview. J Am Med Asoc 1994;272(17):1367–1371.

Chapter 6
Systematic Reviews

Aim

The aim of this chapter is to introduce searching of Medline via PubMed, the use of Boolean operators and the calculation of simple effect measures.

Outcomes

On completing this chapter the reader should be able to undertake a simple search in PubMed using Boolean operators and be able to calculate absolute risk reduction and numbers needed to treat.

Finding and Appraising Systematic Reviews

While the number of Cochrane reviews are increasing steadily, it will be many years before a wide range of dental topics are covered. In addition, because Cochrane reviews focus on the effectiveness of treatment, there are other areas that would benefit from systematic reviews of the available evidence. In this chapter the process of finding and appraising non Cochrane systematic reviews is explained

Consider these scenarios. If you have not already written down your answers to them, do it now before you read the chapter.

Scenario G
A regularly attending patient is having a routine visit six weeks before her wedding. She is interested in whitening her teeth for the big day but she is concerned about the damage it might cause after reading an article in a women's magazine. Because she is so busy with her wedding plans she is interested in doing it at home rather than arranging another appointment.

Scenario H
A patient is keen to follow the advice of her health visitor to breastfeed but has heard that it has been linked to early dental decay. What would you advise?

Scenario G

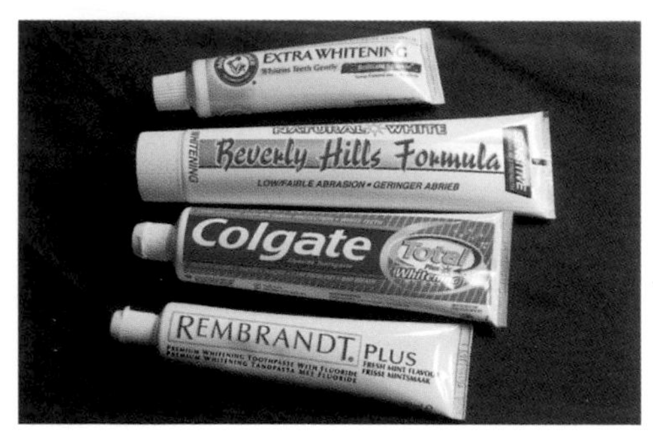

Fig 6-1 Scenario G, home teeth whitening.

A regularly attending patient is having a routine visit six weeks before her wedding. She is interested in whitening her teeth for the big day but is concerned about the damage it might cause after reading an article in a women's magazine. Because she is so busy with her wedding plans she is interested in doing it at home rather than arranging another appointment.

Population	Intervention	Comparison	Outcomes
Adults	Tooth whitening (at home)	Placebo	Change in tooth colour Adverse effects

ASK

The question could be written as:

- In an adult with tooth discolouration would a home tooth whitening kit when compared to placebo improve/change tooth colour?

ACQUIRE

Our first port of call in a search for evidence should be for an evidence-based guideline followed by a search of the Cochrane Library. If there are no reviews on the Cochrane Library the next best place to look for evidence to answer the question is PubMed.

PubMed

PubMed is the USA National Library of Medicine's (NLM) database of biomedical citations and abstracts that is searchable on the internet: (www.pubmed.gov) at no cost.

MEDLINE is the largest component of PubMed and covers over 4800 journals published in the US and more than 70 other countries, primarily from 1966 to the present (see page 117 for further details).

Please note that since preparing this example a Cochrane review on this topic has now been published: Hasson H, Ismail AI, Neiva G. Home-based chemically-induced whitening of teeth in adults. *Cochrane Database of Systematic Reviews* 2006, Issue 4. Art. No.: CD006202. DOI: 10.1002/14651858.CD006202 and the earlier protocol withdrawn.

Searching PubMed: a Step-by-Step Guide to Doing a Simple Search

PubMed is a search engine just like the one in Google. Unlike Google it searches the MEDLINE database for the NLM in the USA.

When you type a word such as *amalgam*, it searches for that word anywhere in its database and shows you the results (Fig 6-2). This type of search is called a *text word search*. It will give you papers in which amalgam (and not necessarily just dental amalgam) may appear in the title or the abstract, but does not necessarily mean the main focus of the paper is amalgam.

Like most reference systems MEDLINE has its own index system. When a biomedical article is added to MEDLINE it is assigned a number of index

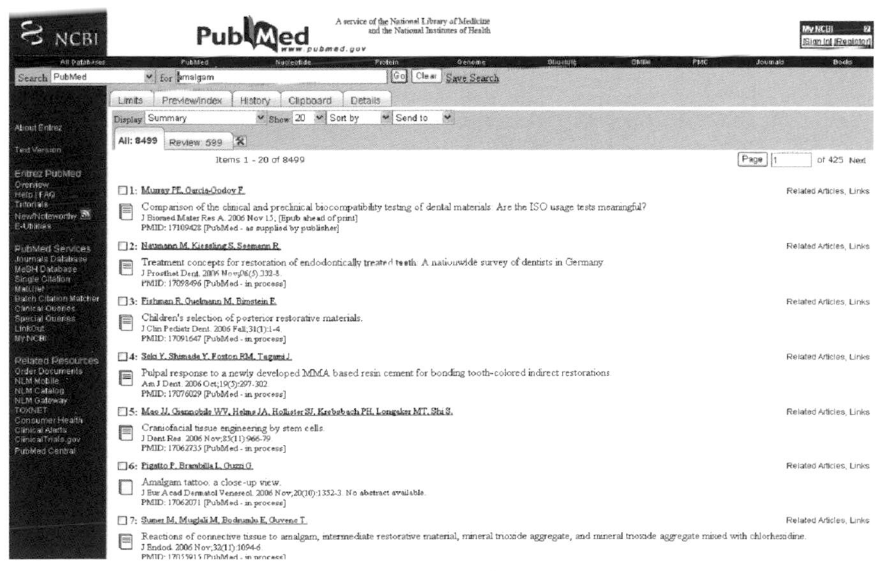

Fig 6-2 PubMed – amalgam text word search.

terms. These index terms are referred to as Medical Subject Heading – MeSH for short.

Selecting MeSH from the dropdown search menu, or the left-hand (blue) column (Fig 6-3), will take you to the MeSH database. Here you can search to see what MeSH terms are used for amalgam. The search actually yields a number of terms but *dental amalgam* is the most suitable. As you can see, this term was introduced to the database in 1965 (Fig 6-4).

Now MEDLINE can be searched using the MeSH term (a MeSH Search). Check the tick box next to the term *dental amalgam* and go to the dropdown box (Fig 6-5) under "send to". Click on "Search box with AND". This will take you to another screen where you can click the search PubMed button to search for *Dental Amalgam* as a MeSH term (Fig 6-6).

Scientific articles are written by humans and MEDLINE is compiled by humans. Consequently if you are conducting a detailed search for information it is best to search the database using both text words and MeSH terms and combining them for each concept in your question. This may take

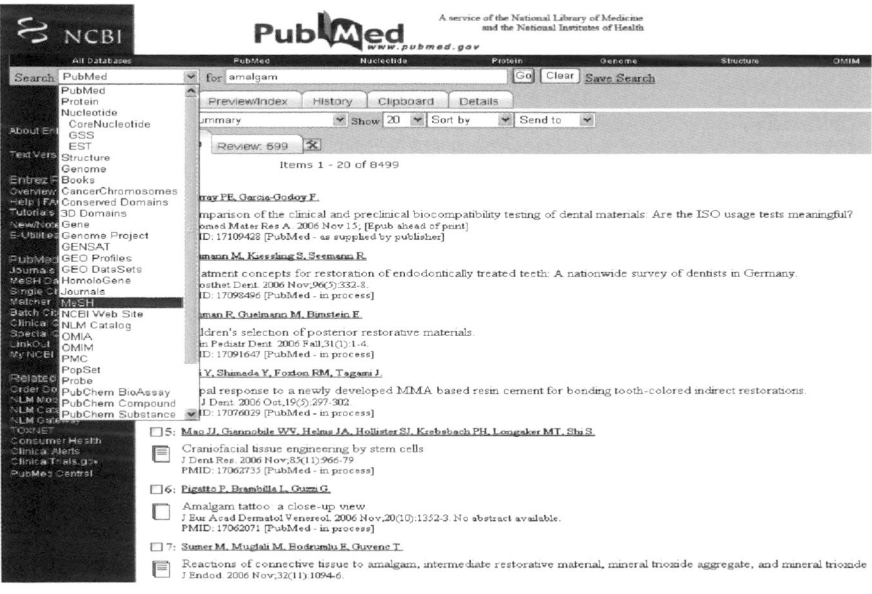

Fig 6-3 PubMed – selecting MeSH.

slightly longer but should help you avoid missing a paper that gives you the right answer to your question.

NCBI

MeSH

A service of the National Library of Medicine
and the National Institutes of Health

All Databases PubMed Nucleotide Protein Genome Structure OMIM

Search MeSH for amalgam Go Clear Save Search

Limits Preview/Index History Clipboard Details

Suggestions: Calgam; Amalcap; Amatine; Amandin; Amanita; Amenta; Amaryl; Algalev; Amazona; Amapor, more...

Display Summary Show 20 Send to

All: 19

Items 1 - 19 of 19

1: Dental Amalgam
An alloy used in restorative dentistry that contains mercury, silver, tin, copper, and possibly zinc.
Year introduced: 1965

2: Amalgam protein, Drosophila [Substance Name]
GenBank M23561
Date introduced: August 8, 2003

3: Agestan [Substance Name]
a low-copper dental amalgam
Date introduced: November 25, 1998

4: silver mercury amalgam [Substance Name]
Date introduced: August 15, 1997

5: Fluor-Alloy [Substance Name]
a fluoride-containing amalgam
Date introduced: September 4, 1996

About Entrez
Text Version
Entrez PubMed
Overview
Help | FAQ
Tutorials
New/Noteworthy
E-Utilities
PubMed Services
Journals Database
MeSH Database
Single Citation Matcher
Batch Citation Matcher
Clinical Queries
Special Queries
LinkOut
My NCBI
Related Resources
Order Documents
NLM Mobile
NLM Catalog
NLM Gateway
TOXNET
Consumer Health

Fig 6-4 PubMed – MeSH amalgam search 1.

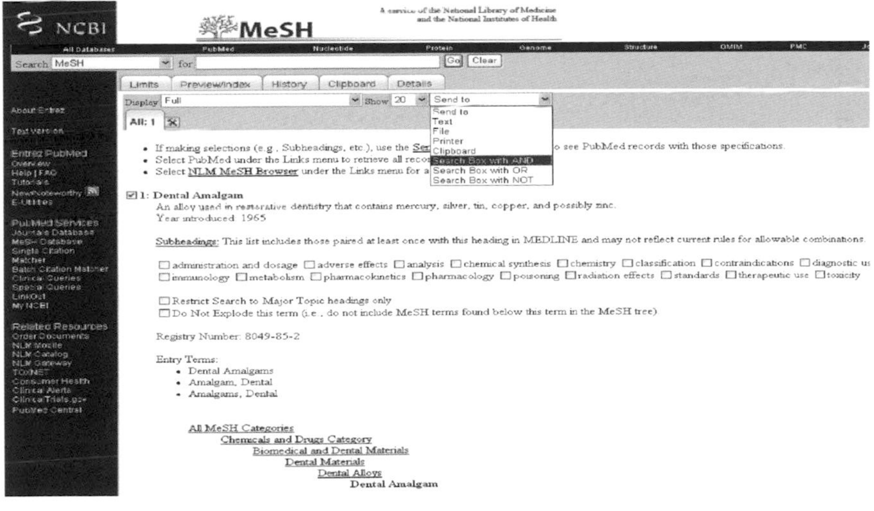

Fig 6-5 PubMed – MeSH amalgam search 2.

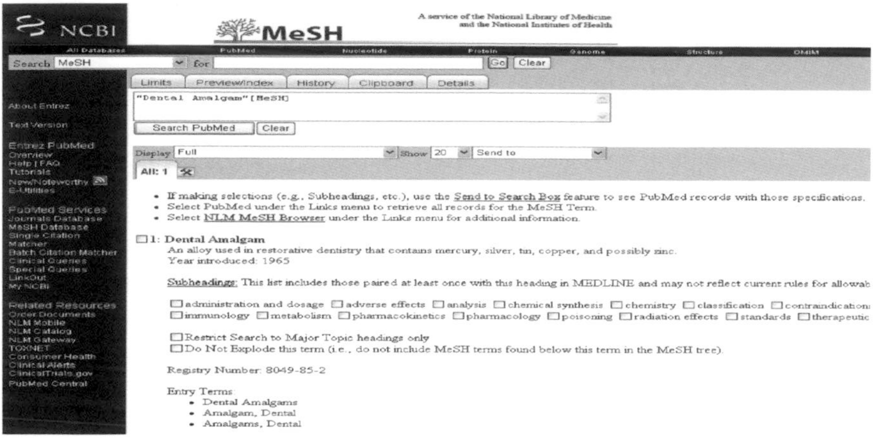

NCBI

MeSH

A service of the National Library of Medicine
and the National Institutes of Health

All Databases | PubMed | Nucleotide | Protein | Genome | Structure | OMIM

Search MeSH for Go Clear

Limits | Preview/Index | History | Clipboard | Details

"Dental Amalgam"[MeSH]

Search PubMed | Clear

Display Full | Show 20 | Send to

All: 1

- If making selections (e.g., Subheadings, etc.), use the Send to Search Box feature to see PubMed records with those specifications.
- Select PubMed under the Links menu to retrieve all records for the MeSH Term.
- Select NLM MeSH Browser under the Links menu for additional information.

1: **Dental Amalgam**

An alloy used in restorative dentistry that contains mercury, silver, tin, copper, and possibly zinc.

Year introduced: 1965

Subheadings: This list includes those paired at least once with this heading in MEDLINE and may not reflect current rules for allowab

administration and dosage | adverse effects | analysis | chemical synthesis | chemistry | classification | contraindication
immunology | metabolism | pharmacokinetics | pharmacology | poisoning | radiation effects | standards | therapeutic

Restrict Search to Major Topic headings only

Do Not Explode this term (i.e., do not include MeSH terms found below this term in the MeSH tree).

Registry Number: 8049-85-2

Entry Terms:

- Dental Amalgams
- Amalgam, Dental
- Amalgams, Dental

About Entrez

Text Version

Entrez PubMed
Overview
Help | FAQ
Tutorials
New/Noteworthy
E-Utilities

PubMed Services
Journals Database
MeSH Database
Single Citation Matcher
Batch Citation Matcher
Clinical Queries
Special Queries
LinkOut
My NCBI

Related Resources
Order Documents
NLM Mobile
NLM Catalog
NLM Gateway
TOXNET
Consumer Health
Clinical Alerts
ClinicalTrials.gov
PubMed Central

Fig 6-6 PubMed – MeSH amalgam search 3.

Combining Terms in PubMed

To combine search terms in PubMed (or any search engine such as Google) you can use the terms AND, OR, NOT and NEAR to tell search engines which keywords you want your results to include or exclude, and whether you require that your keywords appear close to each other.

These words are called Boolean operators after George Boole, an Englishman, who invented them as part of a system of logic in the mid-1800s. For beginners it is best to stick only with the AND and OR terms.

Example

Consider the question:

- In an adult with tooth discolouration would a home tooth whitening kit when compared to placebo improve/change tooth colour?

In the question there are four main themes that can be searched:

- tooth whitening
- at home
- tooth discolouration
- placebo.

Taking each of the themes in turn and searching for both relevant text words and MeSH terms:

Search no.	Search term	Number of references
#1	tooth whitening	1312
#2	tooth bleaching	1281
#3	"tooth bleaching" [MeSH]	1271
#4	#1 OR #2 OR #3	1315

The final search in this sequence #4 uses the Boolean operator OR. This combines all the unique references which appear within these three search terms and produces slightly more references than any of the individual terms (Fig 6-7).

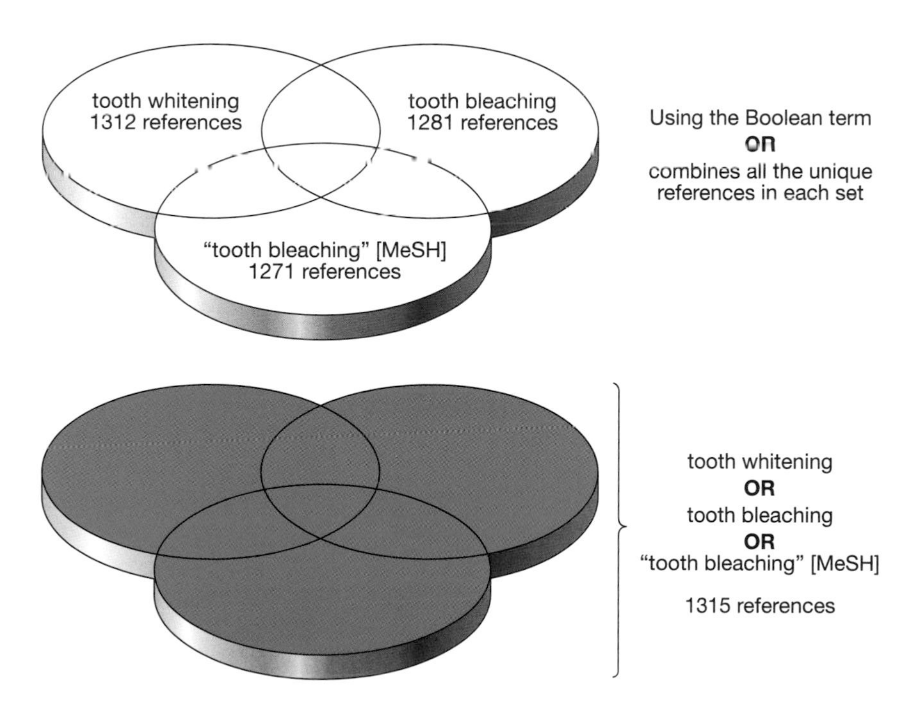

Fig 6-7 Visual representation of use of Boolean operator OR.

Search no.	Search term	Number of references
#5	At home	106,646
#6	Home care	118,648
#7	"dental devices, homecare" [MeSH]	1240
#8	#5 OR #6 OR #7	186,288

Again, search #11 uses the Boolean operator OR; however, on this occasion the combination does not produce any more references than the text word.

Search no.	Search term	Number of references
#9	tooth discolouration	2106
#10	"tooth discolouration" [MeSH]	2087
#11	#9 OR #10	2106

Search no.	Search term	Number of references
#12	Placebo	111,835
#13	"Placebos" [MeSH]	25,576
#14	#12 OR #13	111,835

Now that we have searches for each of our four main themes we can combine them to see if we can find an answer to our question. For searches #15 to #17 we have used the Boolean operator AND. This has reduced the number of references in our searches considerably (see Fig 6-8).

Search no.	Search term	Number of references
#15	#4 (tooth whitening theme) AND #8 (home use theme)	265
#16	#15 AND #11 (tooth discolouration theme)	122
#17	#16 AND (placebo theme)	7

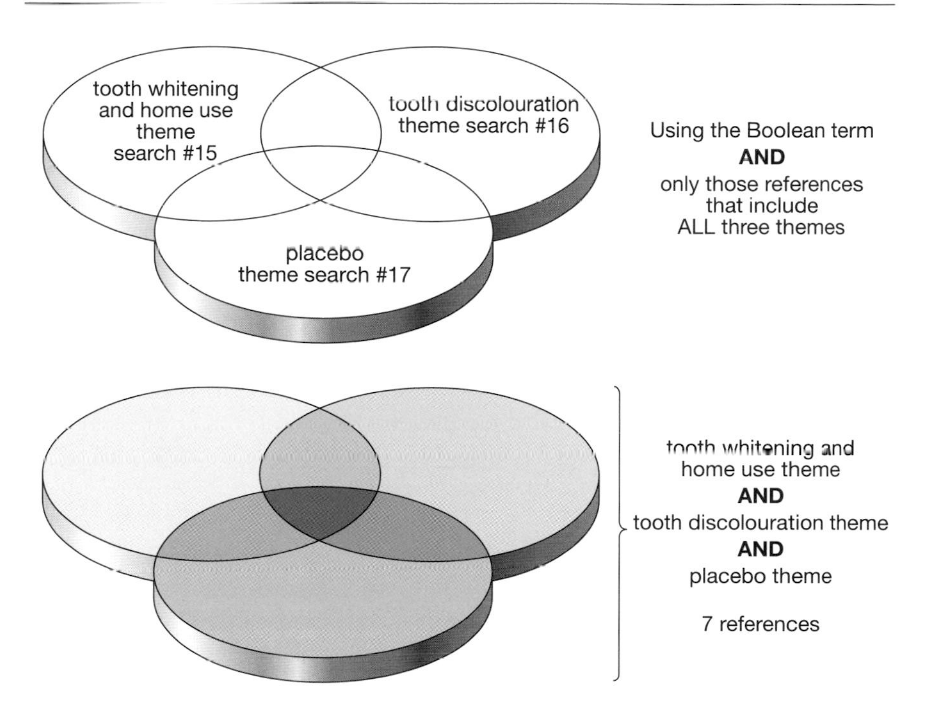

Fig 6-8 Visual representation of use of Boolean operator AND.

When combining searches using Boolean operators it is easy to use AND instead of OR and vice versa, so a useful tip is to think OR means M**OR**E.

Looking through the seven references identified there is one (*Niederman R, Tantraphol MC, Slinin P, Hayes C, Conway S. Effectiveness of dentist-prescribed, home-applied tooth whitening. A meta analysis. J Contemp Dent Pract. 2000 Nov 15;1(4):20-36.*) that seems to address our question directly. A structured abstract (Box 6-1) is available on MEDLINE; and as the *Journal of Contemporary Dental Practice* is freely available electronically, the whole article can be downloaded and appraised. In order to assess the article fully a critical appraisal should be carried out, but the abstract does provide some useful information that we could use if we needed to make a quick decision. (Structured abstracts where methods and results are clearly indicated help. There is information regarding a systematic search with inclusion and exclusion criteria. The results clearly indicate a percentage improvement in the key outcome.)

Box 6-1 **Effectiveness of dentist-prescribed, home-applied tooth whitening: a meta-analysis**

Introduction: Common clinical experience suggests that tooth whitening agents are 100% effective. This study uses meta-analysis of data from published randomised controlled clinical trials to determine the efficacy of tooth whitening agents.

Methods: A MEDLINE search strategy was developed and implemented to systematically identify clinical trials on dentist-prescribed, home-applied tooth whitening agents, using 10% carbamide peroxide, published between 1989 and 1999. Inclusion criteria (e.g. in English, human clinical trials) and exclusion criteria (e.g. not placebo controlled) were established and clinical trials that met these criteria were critically appraised for validity and clinical applicability. Meta-analysis was then used to quantitatively integrate the findings.

Results: Seven studies were identified that met the inclusion and validity criteria. These studies indicated that: Whitening results in a significant mean change of 5.9 shade guide units ($p < 0.01$), while the placebo control group exhibited little change (0.7, 0.6, $p > 0.05$). Some 93% of the bleached patients exhibited two shade guide units of change, while 20% of the placebo control group exhibited this change. The brand of bleaching agent had a significant effect on tooth whitening but the daily application time and duration of treatment did not. Whitening is maintained for six months for half of the people treated. Neither gingival indices nor plaque indices were adversely or favourably affected by bleaching.

Clinical applicability: The data from the reviewed studies indicate that rather than being 100% effective, on average: 73% (93% for bleached group minus 20% placebo group) of people who whiten their teeth will exhibit a whitening that is two shade guide units greater than the placebo. Some 20% of the people who use dentist-prescribed, home-applied bleaching will achieve a mean whitening effect of five shade guide units. Re-treatment for 50% of people may be necessary to maintain this effect longer than six months. The methods used here are internet applicable for other clinical topics.

Niederman R, Tantraphol MC, Slinin P, Hayes C, Conway S. Effectiveness of dentist-prescribed, home-applied tooth whitening. A meta analysis. J Contemp Dent Pract 2000 Nov 15;1(4):20–36.

Finding Systematic Reviews in PubMed Quickly

The process we have outlined above is the basis on which detailed searches for systematic reviews are conducted, albeit the search strategies are much more detailed to ensure no relevant articles are excluded. However, it is possible to identify the same meta-analysis more rapidly using the clinical queries tool in PubMed. This can be found on the left-hand side of PubMed. Clicking on this link brings up a different search page (Fig 6-9); if the term *tooth whitening* is entered in the systematic review search box, 15 studies are identified including the one noted above.

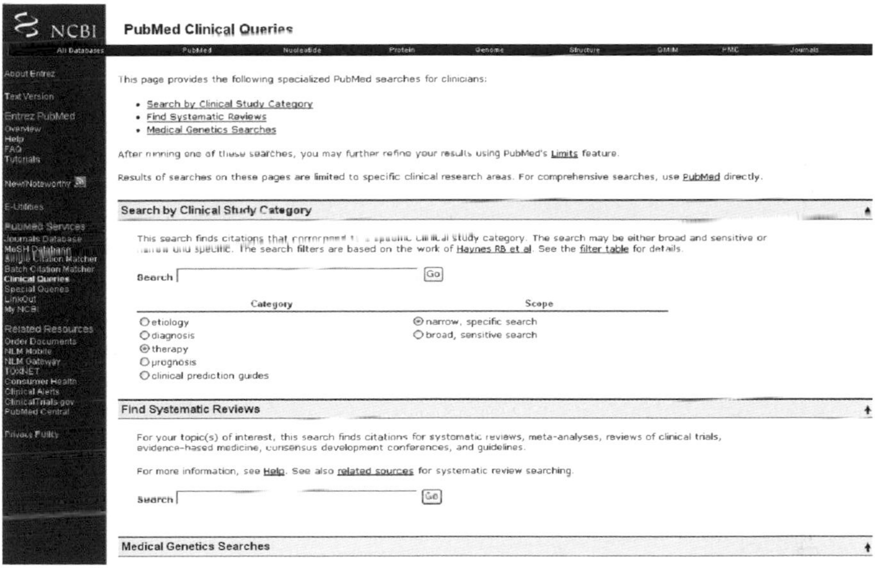

Fig 6-9 PubMed clinical queries page.

APPRAISAL

Appraisal of the full systematic review should be undertaken using a tool such as the CASP systematic review questions (see page 34). The potential benefit (size of the effect) is one of the considerations and this can be presented in several ways. Using the figures given in the abstract (see Box 6-1 and Table 6-1) we describe four of these.

Table 6-1 **Chance of improvement in the test and control group**

	Test (bleach)	Control (placebo)
whitening that is 2 shade guide units greater	93%	20%

What these percentages represent is the risk (chance) of improvement in either the test or control group. There are two simple mathematical methods of expressing the differences between the results in each of these groups: by subtracting them, or presenting them as a ratio.

Subtraction

$$93 - 20 = 73\%$$

The 93% and the 20% represent the risk of improvement in each of the groups so the difference is known as the **Absolute Risk Reduction (ARR)**.

Ratio

$$93/20 = 4.65$$

As we are expressing the risk of improvement in each group, this ratio is known as the **Risk Ratio (RR)**.

If we consider the ARR we can see that there is a big difference between the groups. However, as both groups have improved we need to be aware of what the relative improvement between the groups is. To do this we need to divide the ARR by the risk in the placebo group:

$$(93 - 20)/20 = 3.5$$

This is called the **Relative Risk Reduction (RRR)**.

These three terms are regularly used in clinical studies and should be given along with confidence intervals (see page 72) in reports.

Numbers Needed to Treat

Another way of representing the result is to use the number needed to treat (NNT). This is the inverse of the absolute risk reduction or increase and the number of patients that need to be treated for one to benefit compared with a control. The ideal NNT is 1, where everyone has improved with treatment and no one has improved with control. The higher the NNT, the less effective is the treatment. For our example:

$$\text{NTT} = 100/73 = 1.37$$

In practice this is normally rounded up to the next whole number (as we don't have half a patient) which would give an NNT = 2.

Considering this study we could then say that we would need to treat two patients with a home-whitening product to ensure one patient would see a tooth shade whitening of at least two shade guide units.

Some find this approach more straightforward than others. It is particularly useful to use NNTs when looking to compare two different treatment approaches for the same problem or condition – for example, fissure sealants and topical fluorides for preventing caries. NNTs represent a point estimate for a particular study and should be presented with confidence intervals with due consideration being paid to the circumstances of the study.

APPLY

In terms of answering our patient's question, we can use the identified paper to reassure her that a *10% carbamide peroxide* product could be expected to whiten her tooth colour by at least two shades. We could even give her some indication with a shade guide. We could also indicate that some patients (one in five) could achieve a five-shade improvement. In terms of negative effects, the paper does not indicate adverse effects other than the fact that the improvement in shade is not maintained and one in two patients may require re-treatment in order to maintain the effect at six months.

Scenario H

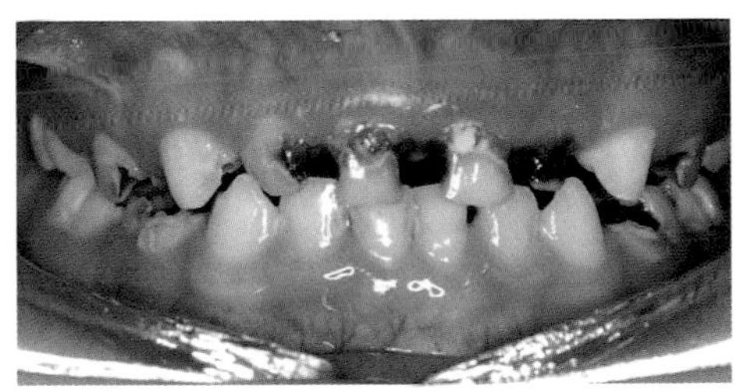

Fig 6-10 Scenario H, breastfeeding and caries.

A patient is keen to follow the advice of her health visitor to breastfeed but has heard that it has been linked to early dental decay. What would you advise?

Population	Intervention	Comparison	Outcomes
Children	Breast feeding	Bottle fed	Increased caries

The question is straightforward:
- Is breastfeeding linked to an increase in dental caries?

ACQUIRE

Using the clinical tools link on the home page of PubMed (Fig 6-9), the key search terms for this question "breastfeeding" and "dental caries" are entered into the systematic reviews search box and the return key or go buttons pressed. The search identifies five reviews, two of which address the question under consideration:

- *Ribeiro NM, Ribeiro MA. [Breastfeeding and early childhood caries: a critical review] J Pediatr (Rio J) 2004 Nov;80(5 Suppl):S199–210. Portuguese.*
- *Valaitis R, Hesch R, Passarelli C, Sheehan D, Sinton J. A systematic review of the relationship between breastfeeding and early childhood caries. Can J Public Health 2000 Nov–Dec;91(6):411–7.*

The Ribeiro review is the most recent. If you click on the title it takes you to the abstract page and you will see that, although the reference indicated that it is in Portuguese, a free full-text version is available to download in English (www.jped.com.br/conteudo/04-80-S199/ing.asp). With the full-text version of the paper you are in a position to appraise the article.

APPRAISE and APPLY

A basic appraisal of the full article is shown in Table 6-2.

If the review is well conducted, it is always the last question of the appraisal tool above that is the most important. This is because it is the next stage of

Table 6-2 **Basic appraisal of breastfeeding and early childhood caries: a critical review** (continued over page)

Did the review ask a clearly focused question?	As with many studies, the objective of the review is much more clearly stated in the abstract than in the body of the text but the focus is the investigation of a possible relationship between breastfeeding and caries.
Did the review include the right type of study?	The types of study included in the review have not been clearly specified. The majority of included studies have been defined as cross-sectional studies. Randomised controlled trials, while feasible, may not be practical or ethical in this group, so a prospective cohort would be the most appropriate design to answer the question.

Table 6-2 **Basic appraisal of breastfeeding and early childhood caries: a critical review** (continued)

Did the reviewers try to identify all relevant studies?	Three databases, MEDLINE (see page 117), LILACS (see page 118) and The Scientific Electronic Library Online (SciELO – an electronic library covering a selected collection of Brazilian scientific journals) were searched as well as the references of the identified articles.
Did the reviewers assess the quality of the included studies?	There appears to be no formal quality assessment of the articles, and the description of the reviews methodology is limited.
If the results of the studies have been combined, was it reasonable to do so?	A qualitative summary of the findings has been presented, but there is no indication of inclusion and exclusion criteria so it is difficult to assess. As noted the majority of the studies are cross-sectional.
How are the results presented and what is the main result?	A qualitative summary.
How precise are these results?	Not applicable as no quantitative data presented.
Can the results be applied to the local population?	The included studies come from a wide range of countries so it seems reasonable for these to be used locally.
Were all important outcomes considered?	Yes.
Should policy or practice change as a result of the evidence contained in this review?	The authors concluded: "*there is no scientific evidence that confirms that breast milk is associated with caries development*".

the evidence-based method, namely the application point; that is, should I use it in my practice? If you read the review in full you will see (hopefully) that there are some limitations in the methodology of the review and the papers that were included. Consequently the authors' conclusion seems to overinterpret the evidence presented.

A number of studies have been conducted since the review in 2000 by Valaitis et al. (2000), in which they noted:

"A lack of methodological consistency related to the study of the association of breastfeeding and ECC, and inconsistent definitions of ECC and breastfeeding, make it difficult to draw conclusions. Moderate articles indicate that breastfeeding for over one year and at night beyond eruption of teeth may be associated with ECC. Due to conflicting findings in less rigorous research studies, no definitive time at which an infant should be weaned was determined, and parents should begin an early and consistent mouth care regime."

Taking both reviews into account we can probably say that there is some evidence that breastfeeding is *not* associated with caries development. A small number of studies of low quality have linked prolonged *ad libitum* and nocturnal breastfeeding to early childhood caries. However, further high-quality studies are needed to address this question.

In terms of advice to the new mum, she should be advised to breastfeed as advised by her health visitors. This is because there is extensive evidence for short- and long-term health benefits of breastfeeding, with the World Health Organization recommending that all infants should be fed exclusively on breast milk from birth to six months of age (World Health Organization, 2002). Mum should also be encouraged to clean her child's teeth regularly and consistently as soon as the first tooth erupts.

Key Points

- Tools are available to identify systematic reviews quickly on PubMed.
- A wide range of systematic reviews is available which can provide good evidence for clinical practice.
- The quality of systematic reviews varies widely so they need to be critically appraised before applying in clinical practice.
- Summaries of systematic reviews are available from a number of websites (see page 119) and secondary journals.

References

Valaitis R, Hesch R, Passarelli C, Sheehan D, Sinton J. A systematic review of the relationship between breastfeeding and early childhood caries. Can J Public Health 2000;91(6):411–417.

World Health Organization. Infant and young child nutrition; global strategy for infant and young child feeding. Geneva: WHO, 2002. Executive Board paper. Report No. EB 109/12 2002.

Chapter 7

Individual Studies

Aim

The aim of this chapter is to show which types of study are needed to answer particular questions, outline some hints for searching, and introduce the basic questions to address in critical appraisal.

Outcomes

On completion of this chapter the reader will be able to identify the most appropriate study design to answer questions, and be aware of the three basic questions to address in a critical appraisal.

Using Individual Studies

If there are no evidence-based guidelines, Cochrane reviews or other systematic reviews to address our clinical problems then we must look to individual studies.

What Type of Study?

The type of study that we need to look for depends on the question that we need answered (see Table 7-1).

Let us consider examples of the main question types:

- What is the best type of restoration for carious primary molar teeth?
- What is the best method of preventing root caries in adult patients?
- What are the side-effects of using chlorhexidine mouthwash for the treatment of periodontal disease?
- Are digital x-ray systems better at diagnosing caries than film-based systems?
- Are school-based toothbrushing programmes cost-effective?
- What are teenagers' reasons for undergoing orthodontic treatment?

Table 7-1 **What is the most appropriate study design to answer the question?**

Clinical problem	Most appropriate study design
Treatment/prevention, aetiology	RCT
Prognosis	Individual inception cohort study with ≥ 80% follow-up
Diagnosis	Validating cohort study with good reference standards
Differential diagnosis/ symptom prevalence study	Prospective cohort study with good follow-up
Economic and decision analyses	Analysis based on clinically sensible costs or alternatives; systematic review(s) of the evidence; and including multi-way sensitivity analyses
Acceptability, appropriateness and quality of care, reasons for undergoing treatment	Qualitative studies

ASK

As before, you need to develop a PICO question for each of these questions (Table 7-2).

ACQUIRE

We now need to find out whether there are any studies to answer these questions. We will assume for the moment that there are no evidence-based guidelines, Cochrane or other systematic reviews available to answer our questions. This means that the starting-point for our search is the PubMed database.

To begin the search we should use a combination of free text and MeSH searches as described in Chapter 6 for each of the questions. Once you have developed the key themes of your searches you can then combine them using the Boolean terms AND and OR. (See the Appendix for example searches for each of the questions above.)

Table 7-2 **PICO questions**

Question	Patient	Intervention	Comparison	Outcome
What is the best type of restoration for carious primary molar teeth?	Child with carious teeth	Amalgam, composite, compomer, glass-ionomers, pre-formed metal crown, extraction, no-restoration	Amalgam, composite, compomer, glass-ionomers, pre-formed metal crown, extraction, no-restoration	No pain, no swelling, no infection, tooth survival to exfoliation
What is the best method of preventing root caries in adult patients?	Adult at risk of root caries	Topical fluorides, restorations, diet modification, chlorhexidine mouthwash	Topical fluorides, restorations, diet modification, chlorhexidine mouthwash	Caries
What are the side-effects of using chlorhexidine mouthwash for the treatment of periodontal disease?	Adults with periodontal disease	Chlorhexidine mouthwash	Placebo	Staining, altered taste
Are digital x-ray systems better at diagnosing caries than film-based systems?	All patients requiring dental x-rays	Digital x-ray	Film-based x-ray systems	Improved diagnosis, increased sensitivity and specificity
Are school-based toothbrushing programmes cost-effective?	School-aged children	Toothbrushing programmes	No programme	Cost effectiveness
What are teenagers' reasons for undergoing orthodontic treatment?	Children requiring orthodontic treatment	Orthodontic treatment		Improved compliance

The searches will give us a large number of studies to consider. However, we know that for treatment and prevention questions the best type of study to give us a definite answer is a randomised controlled trial.

We could look through the complete list of references that we find in our individual question search in PubMed for all the randomised controlled trials. If our search has identified a lot of references this could take us a long time. Fortunately PubMed has a way of speeding up the process.

PubMed Limits

If the "limits tab" is clicked it provides a range of options to enable us to limit our search (Fig 7-1). Some of the more useful options are:

- abstracts (articles with abstracts tend to be of higher quality)
- human (versus animal)
- language (whatever languages you are comfortable reading)
- type of article.

However there are more options that are useful in specific circumstances. (It is worth noting that once the limits button is clicked it stays clicked and

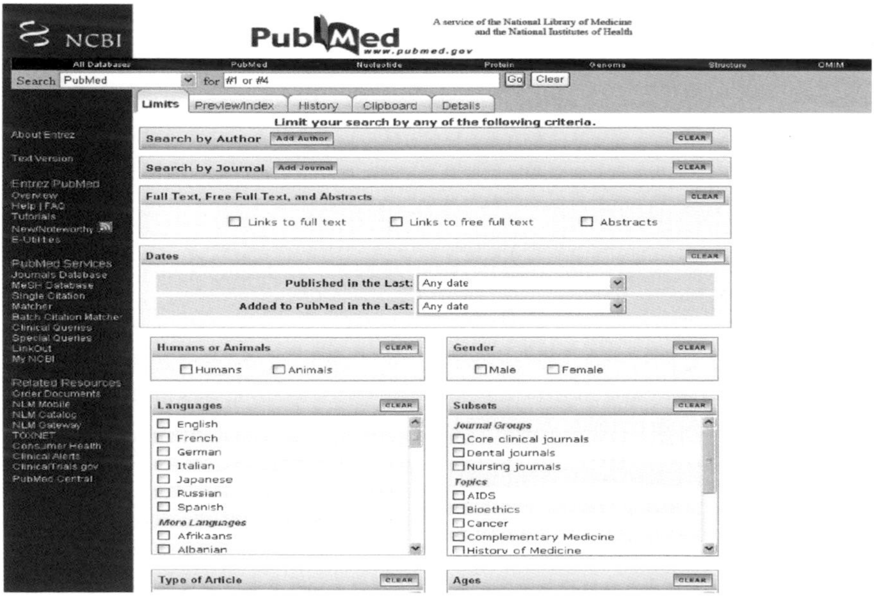

Fig 7-1 PubMed limits page.

all subsequent searches have the limits that you have chosen imposed unless you unclick the limits tab.)

Under the "type of article" box you will see that there is a tick box for randomised controlled trials. Ticking this and pressing the return key will limit your search to randomised controlled trials. While this filter will pick up most randomised controlled trials, it will not pick up all of them and specific search filters have been developed. More information on search filters can be found at www.shef.ac.uk/scharr/ir/filter.html.

APPRAISE

We have seen previously a list of questions (CASP appraisal tools) to help decide whether guidelines and systematic reviews are worth using. Similar questions/tools exist for other studies types. The questions included within each of these tools vary with the study designs. However, whatever the tools, they are helping you to answer three basic questions about the study:
- is it valid?
- what are the results?
- are the results relevant to my problem?

Validity

Validity has two elements:
- *Internal validity* – which can be seen as the degree to which the results of a study are likely to approximate to the "truth" for the circumstances being studied.
- *External validity* – the degree to which the effects observed in the study are applicable to the outside world.

Results

It is deciding what the results of the study are that causes most concern to most people undertaking appraisal. This is because some understanding of mathematics and basic statistical terms is required. A detailed understanding of statistics is not required to appraise the majority of studies and the simple calculations presented in this book will assist you in understanding them.

Relevance

This is often the key issue for clinicians and the one element that they are usually happiest with. If the study is valid and the results clear then a decision as to whether it is appropriate for them to use in their own practice is one that they are comfortable in making.

In the following chapters we will deal with the key elements in appraising and understanding the results of:

- randomised controlled trials
- cohort studies
- diagnostic tests
- qualitative studies.

Key Points

First identify the most appropriate study design to answer your clinical question.

Then consider:

- is it valid?
- what are the results?
- are the results relevant to my problem?

Chapter 8

Study Appraisal: Randomised Controlled Trials

Aim

The aim of this chapter is to outline the key elements of randomised controlled trials (RCTs) together with how to appraise an RCT, introduce the CONSORT statement and how to calculate simple measures of effect.

Outcomes

On completion of this chapter readers will understand the key features of an RCT and have 10 questions with which to appraise an RCT. They will also be able to calculate simple measures of effect.

What is an RCT?

The RCT is one of the simplest, most powerful tools of research. In essence, the RCT is a study in which people are allocated at random to receive one of several clinical interventions. In its simplest form it can be used to compare two treatments (see Fig 8-1).

Randomised controlled trials are the most rigorous way of determining whether a cause-and-effect relationship exists between treatment and outcome and for assessing the cost-effectiveness of a treatment.

RCTs are the best study design to answer questions related to therapy, prevention, aetiology and harm. Key elements of good RCTs are:

- Good randomisation procedures (allocation concealment).
- Patients masked (blinded) to whether they receive the test treatment or the control treatment.
- Clinicians masked (blinded) to whether their patients receive the test treatment or the control treatment.
- All participants followed up to the end of the study.
- All participants analysed in the groups to which they were randomised (intention to treat).

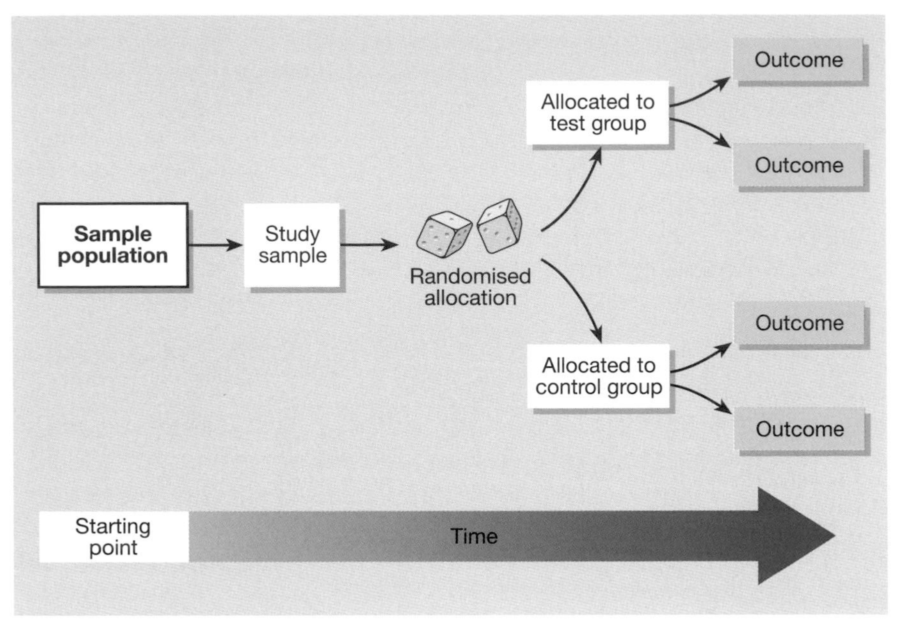

Fig 8-1 Randomised controlled trials.

The majority of tools available to appraise RCTs focus on helping the appraiser determine whether the key elements of RCTs mentioned above are present. A good example of one of these tools is available from the CASP website. The questions in the tool are derived from papers by Guyatt et al. (1993, 1994). See Fig 8-2.

Is the Study Clearly Focused?

This question is to help clarify whether the researchers have developed a clear research question. The process of developing a research question should be similar to the process you have been through to help develop your clear clinical questions. Consequently the study could have been investigating a clearly defined population (e.g. adults with rapidly progressing periodontal disease), comparing specific treatment (e.g. root planing and antimicrobial treatment versus root planing alone) or looking at clear outcomes. These outcomes may be clinical outcomes such as pocket depth, bleeding on probing or tooth or attachment loss, or patient-relevant outcomes such as pain, discomfort, or quality-of-life measures.

	Yes	No	Can't tell
1. Did the study ask a clearly-focused question?	☐	☐	☐
2. Was this a randomised controlled trial and was it appropriately so?	☐	☐	☐
3. Were participants appropriately allocated to intervention and control groups?	☐	☐	☐
4. Were participants, staff and study personnel "masked" to participants' study group?	☐	☐	☐
5. Were all of the participants who entered the trial accounted for at its conclusion?	☐	☐	☐
6. Were the participants in all groups followed up and data collected in the same way?	☐	☐	☐
7. Did the study have enough participants to minimise the play of chance?	☐	☐	☐
8. How are the results presented, and what is the main result?	----------------		
9. How precise are these results?	----------------		
10. Were all important outcomes considered so that the results can be applied?	☐	☐	☐

Fig 8-2 CASP 10 questions to appraise a randomised controlled trial.

Is it a Randomised Controlled Trial?

You need to be clear that the trial was randomised and that a randomised controlled trial was the appropriate study design to answer the question.

The first two questions are designed to be screening questions. *If you answer "no" to these first two questions there is likely to be little gained from reading the paper.*

The remaining questions address the key elements of RCTs in more detail.

Were Participants Appropriately Allocated?

Randomisation is the only way to control for confounders that are not known or not measured in the study; therefore we need to know if the process of allocation of participants to the intervention and control groups was properly random. The best way of achieving this is to ensure the process is conducted by someone who is not recruiting patients, for example a central office. Good methods of randomisation are computer-generated random number sequences or random number tables.

In some cases, for example in a periodontal study, you may wish to separate out smokers and non-smokers before randomisation (stratification), to ensure a balance of smokers and non-smokers in the intervention and control groups.

With robust randomisation procedures you would expect there to be a balance of characteristics between the groups at baseline and for these to be discussed in the paper. You should consider whether any baseline differences would affect the outcome.

Were Participants, Staff and Study Personnel "Masked" to Participants' Study Group?

If you are involved in testing a new material or treatment you are likely to have an opinion on whether or not it works. In some cases those conducting the study will have been involved in developing the material or treatment. Whatever role you may or may not have had, however balanced you think that you are, you will have a bias as to whether or not you think the material/treatment will work.

Consequently it is important that as many as possible of those involved in the trial are masked. This is not always possible; for example, two filling materials under test may be obviously different in colour. Being able to mask the individual assessing the outcome is key, if possible, as is being able to mask the patients.

Were All of the Participants who Entered the Trial Accounted for at its Conclusion?

In an ideal world all the patients who entered the trial at the beginning would complete the trial, all those assigned to the intervention under study would have received it, and all those in the control group would have received that option. Unfortunately things in real life are never that simple. It is not unusual for people to drop out of studies and on occasion for some to get the control option when they have been allocated to the intervention option and vice versa.

When participants drop out of a trial this is referred to as loss to follow-up. Loss to follow-up can have a significant effect on the study and investigators usually make strenuous efforts to ensure this is minimised. From an appraisal perspective it is important to know how many drop out in each group as this can have an important bearing on the result. If the authors have followed the CONSORT (Consolidated Standards of Reporting Trials) recommendations, which offer a standard method for the reporting of trials, these will be detailed in a flow chart (see Fig 8-3). More information about CONSORT can be found at www.consort-statement.org/ index.html.

Were the Participants in All Groups Followed Up and Data Collected in the Same Way?

What you are looking for here is whether both intervention and control groups were followed up at the same time, and whether they received the

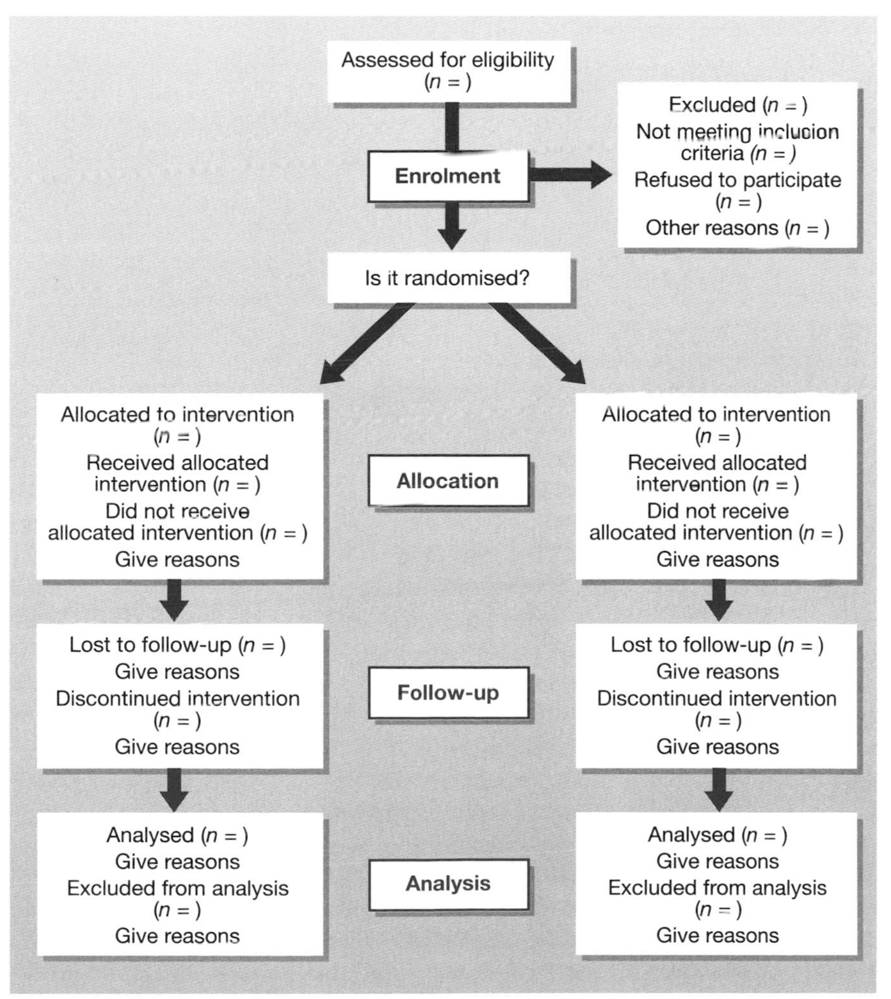

Fig 8-3 Consort flow chart.

same amount of attention from the researchers or healthcare workers. If there were any differences, you have to consider if this has any likely impact on the outcomes being looked at.

For example, if you were comparing two different interventions for treating periodontal disease over a period of 12 months and one group had treatment A and a follow-up at 6 and 12 months whereas the other group had treatment B but were followed up every month, it is important to realise that the regular monthly visits are likely to have a reinforcing effect over and above the effect of the difference, if any, between treatments A and B.

Did the Study Have Enough Participants to Minimise the Play of Chance?
Why is this important? If we consider a trial where we compare two treatments R and Q there are four possible outcomes (Table 8-1): two where the trial confirms the truth and two where the answer is in error.

Table 8-1 **Possible outcomes of a trial**

		The truth	
		R is better than Q	R is no better than Q
The trial shows	R is better than Q	✓	✗
	R is no better than Q	✗	✓

When the trial shows that treatment R is better than treatment Q when it is not, this is a called a **type I error** (a false positive). The consequence of this could be to allow an ineffective treatment to be performed.

When the trial shows that treatment R is no better than treatment Q when it actually is, this is called a **type II error** (a false negative). Consider a new drug that will be put on the market if we can show that it is better than a placebo. The consequence here could be to prevent or delay the introduction of an effective treatment.

To avoid a type II error a study needs to have a sample that is big enough to detect a difference. To decide whether a study is big enough you should look to see if a power calculation has been performed. This provides an estimate of the number of participants necessary to show a difference. Power is formally defined as the chance of detecting a specified difference (or effect size) if one exists; it is usually set at 80% (alternatively this can be thought of as a 20% (1 in 5) chance of missing a difference if one exists). The smaller the change or effect you are looking for the larger the sample size needs to be.

How Are the Results Presented, and What is the Main Result?

What you are looking for here is whether the authors have reported any differences in the outcomes between the groups. Further, how they have expressed this – for example, percentages, relative risks, or survival curves – if they have provided a clear bottom line result for the study. You also need to consider the size of the result and how clinically meaningful it is. If several outcomes are provided it is useful to concentrate on the one you find most relevant to your clinical practice.

It is useful to construct a table, as shown in Table 8-2, to help you identify the relevant result. Using this type of table you can calculate simple measures of effectiveness, risk, relative risks, absolute risk reduction and numbers needed to treat as shown on pages 53–55.

Table 8-2 **Key elements of information needed to help you measure effects**

	Test group	**Control group**
Participants at start		
Drop-outs		
Number with outcome of interest		

Example

In the paper *Baysan A, Lynch E, Ellwood R, Davies R, Petersson L, Borsboom P. Reversal of primary root caries using dentifrices containing 5,000 and 1,100 ppm fluoride. Caries Res 2001;35(1):41-46*, the following quotes provide the information needed to complete the table.

"At baseline, 107 subjects (130 lesions) were recruited into the 5,000 ppm F–group. Of these 2 subjects failed to attend for either the 3- or 6-month examination, 1 chose to withdraw from the study, 1 had the affected tooth extracted and 1 subject had missing data. Of the 94 subjects (132 lesions) recruited into the 1,100 ppm F–group, 5 failed to attend for examination, 1 withdrew, 2 had the affected teeth filled and 2 had missing data.

At 6 months, 58 (56.9%) of the subjects using the 5,000 ppm F–dentifrice and 24 (28.6%) using the 1,100 ppm F–dentifrice had 1 or more lesions that had become hard (p = 0.002)." (Table 8-3)

Table 8-3 **Dentifrices containing 5000 and 1100 ppm fluoride**

	Test group *(5000 ppm)*	**Control group** *(1100 ppm)*
Participants at start	107	94
Drop-outs	2	5
Number with outcome of interest	58	24

Chance (risk) of improving in test group	= 58/107	= 54.2%*
Chance (risk) of improving in control group	= 24/94	= 25.5%*
Absolute risk reduction	= 54.2 – 25.5	= 28.7%
Risk ratio	= 54.2/25.5	= 2.12
Relative risk reduction	= (54.2 – 25.5)/25.2	= 1.13
Numbers needed to treat	= 100/28.7	= 3.48 (4)

*Data differ slightly from those presented in the original paper as an intention-to-treat approach has been taken.

How Precise Are These Results?

Here we are hoping and expecting that the researchers have provided confidence intervals (CIs) for their results (see page 132).

Confidence intervals

If we wanted to know the average height of the adult male population (18- to 64-year-olds) of the UK, the only way we would know exactly would be to measure every male in this age group. Clearly measuring several million people's height is impossible, so we would take a sample. From this sample (say 3000) we would calculate the average (mean) height, e.g. 177.69 cm

(5 ft 10 in.); we could also calculate a confidence interval. Typically a 95% CI is calculated but sometimes a 99% level is used (in our example this might be 95% CI 173.9 to190.5 cm or 5 ft 8 in. to 6 ft 3 in.).

What this means is that for the case of 95% CI we are 95% certain (i.e. 1 in 20 chance of being wrong) that the average height for the adult male population (aged 18–64) lies between 173.9 cm and 190.5 cm. So the CI represents how good our estimate of male height is, and the narrower the limits the more precise our estimate.

So in appraising a study, what we are looking for are narrow confidence intervals.

***p*-values**

Most research involves making a hypothesis and then collecting data to test that hypothesis. Researchers will usually establish a null hypothesis, i.e. one that presumes that there will be no difference (no effect) as a result of the treatment.

A *p*-value is a measure of how much evidence we have against the null hypothesis. The smaller the *p*-value, the more evidence we have against the null hypothesis. It is also a measure of how likely we are to get a certain sample result or a result "more extreme", assuming the null hypothesis is true.

It is customary to reject a hypothesis if the *p*-value is less than 0.05, but sometimes researchers will use a stricter cut-off (e.g. 0.01).

Consider how often you would see a similar result by chance, when actually there was no effect by the drug or treatment. There are potentially two extremes: that this was impossible or that it was absolutely certain that it would happen. If we draw a line running from 0 to 1 where 0 represents impossible and 1 absolutely certain, then at a point halfway along the line we would be in balance (50/50), not knowing whether the treatment has an effect or not (Fig 8-4). (This is the same as the effect occurring by chance.) As the line runs from 0 to 1 this could be represented as 0.5.

If we now consider where we would place the *p*-value of 0.05 on the line, this is much nearer the impossible end of the line and represents a 1 in 20 chance that the result could have occurred by chance. Consequently a *p*-value of 0.01 is even nearer the impossible end, representing a 1 in 100 possibility that the result could have occurred by chance.

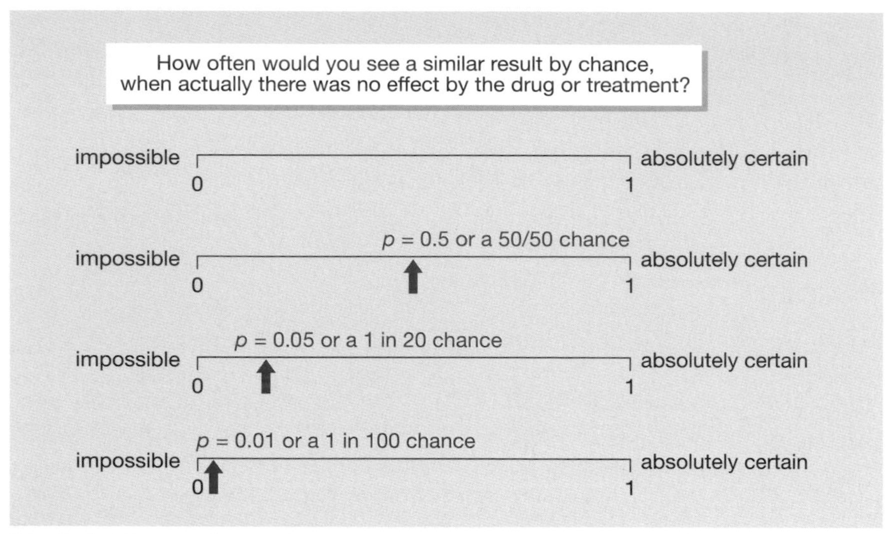

Fig 8-4 Chance observation.

Were All Important Outcomes Considered So the Results Can Be Applied?
As an individual practitioner you will be most concerned about whether important outcomes that affect you and your patient will have been considered. Therefore you need to consider if the participants in the trial were so different from your patients or the ones you see regularly in your practice that you would **not** be able to apply the results locally.

Other issues to consider are whether any benefit reported outweighs any harms and/ or costs of adopting the treatments or interventions considered. They might not be available for the study but you may be able to get them from elsewhere.

Finally, if you believe the results and are happy, you need to consider how you will change your practice as a result. This could be simply change in use of a dental material, participating in a course to learn a new treatment technique or purchasing of new equipment. If you do decide to change, it may also be worth considering auditing your outcomes to see if the changes you make give you the same improvements as described in the paper.

Key Points

- For most intervention or treatment studies, a randomised controlled trial is the highest level of evidence (barring systematic reviews and guidelines).

- Not all clinical trials are created equally. A simple 10-question tool is available for the appraisal of randomised controlled trials. This is available from www.phru.nhs.uk/Pages/PHD/resources.htm.
- If you agree with the findings in the papers you appraise, you should consider changing the way you practise for that clinical situation, if appropriate for your patients.

References

Guyatt GH, Sackett DL, Cook DJ. Users' guides to the medical literature. II. How to use an article about therapy or prevention. A. Are the results of the study valid? Evidence-Based Medicine Working Group. J Am Med Assoc 1993;270(21):2598–601.

Guyatt GH, Sackett DL, Cook DJ. Users' guides to the medical literature. II. How to use an article about therapy or prevention. B. What were the results and will they help me in caring for my patients? Evidence-Based Medicine Working Group. J Am Med Assoc 1994;271(1):59–63.

Moher D, Schulz KF, Altman DG. The CONSORT statement: revised recommendations for improving the quality of reports of parallel-group randomised trials. Lancet 2001;357(9263):1191–1194.

Additional Reading

ASSERT – A standard for the scientific and ethical review of trials. www.assert-statement.org/.

CONSORT – checklist and flow diagram to improve the quality of reports of randomized controlled trials. www.consort-statement.org/.

Greenhalgh T. How to read a paper: getting your bearings (deciding what the paper is about). Br Med J 1997;315:243–246.

Jadad, AR. Randomised Controlled Trials. London: BMJ Books, 1998.

Plint AC, Moher D, Morrison A, Schulz K, Altman DG, Hill C, Gaboury I. Does the CONSORT checklist improve the quality of reports of randomised controlled trials? A systematic review. Med J Aust 2006;185(5):263–267.
Sutherland SE. Evidence-based dentistry: Part V. Critical appraisal of the dental literature: papers about therapy. J Can Dent Assoc 2001;67(8):442–445. www.cda-adc.ca/jcda/vol-67/issue-8/442.html.

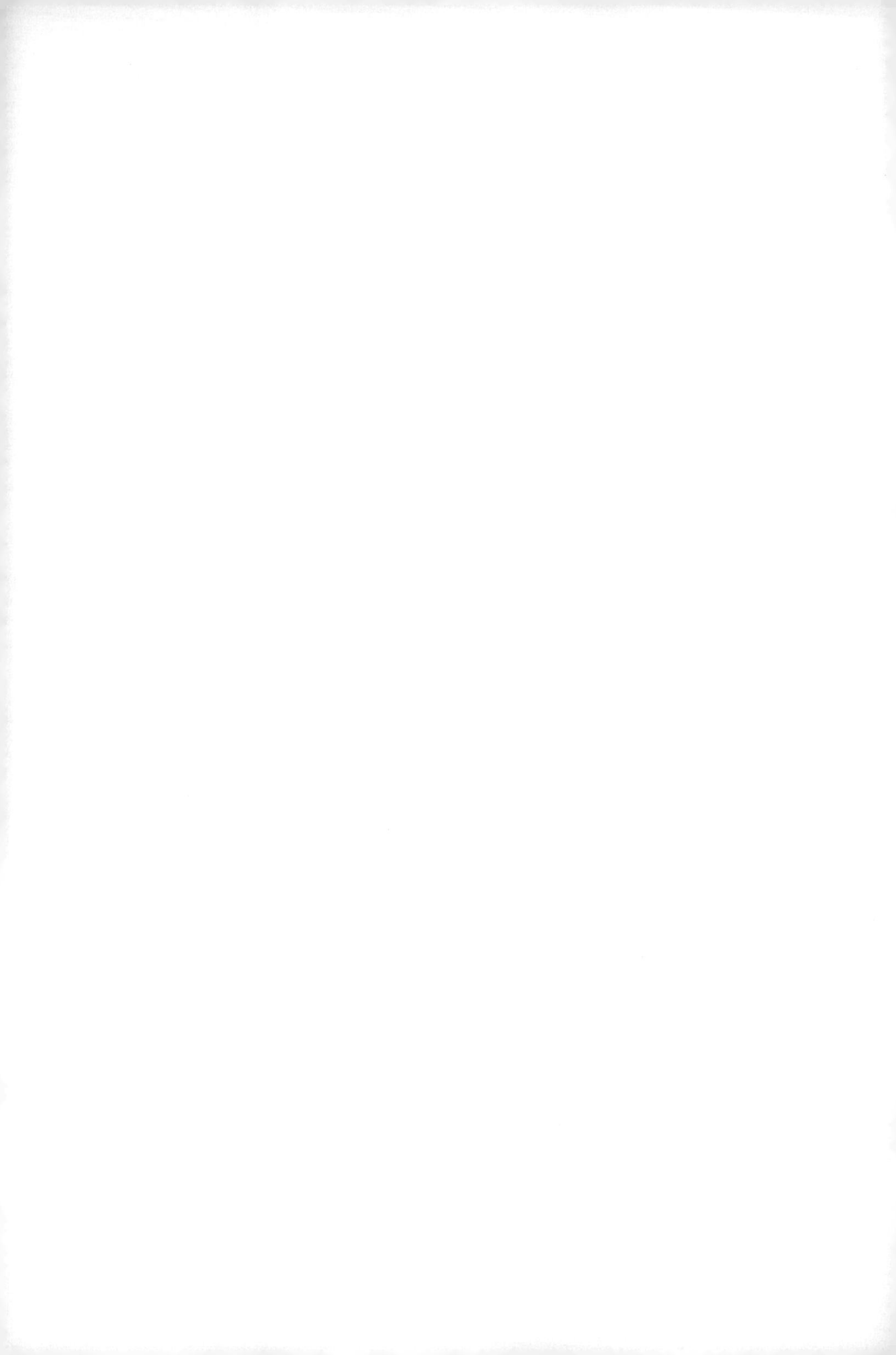

Chapter 9

Study Appraisal: Cohort Studies

Aim

This aim of this chapter is to outline how to appraise a cohort study, explain what risk and odds ratios are and show how to calculate them.

Outcomes

On completion of this chapter the reader should understand the key differences between RCT and cohort studies and have a list of questions to be able to appraise a cohort study.

What Is a Cohort Study?

A cohort study is an observational study; it differs from a clinical trial in that the researchers are not directly trying to treat or prevent a disease or condition. A cohort study is one in which a group of participants is studied over time (Fig 9-1). The group can be selected to represent a population of interest (e.g. smokers, patients with oral lichen planus or leukoplakia), or they could be a group of individuals linked in some way, for example a birth cohort (all those born during a particular period), a disease, education or employment. Participants are followed over time and data are collected on health outcomes and/or exposure to risk factors. A cohort study can be either prospective or retrospective.

Randomised controlled trials are considered the best method for providing evidence on efficacy. However, they are criticised for focusing on highly selected patients and outcomes, and are subject to ethical and logistical constraints (Black, 1996). Cohort studies can address some of these issues, evaluating larger groups of diverse individuals over long periods with the possibility of providing information on a range of outcomes and possibly rare events. While cohort studies have potential to provide useful evidence, concerns regarding the validity of evidence derived from them have been raised. A comparison with randomised controlled studies is shown in Table 9-1 on page 79. In terms of appraising cohort studies CASP provides a similar tool to that available for randomised controlled trials (Fig 9-2 on page 80).

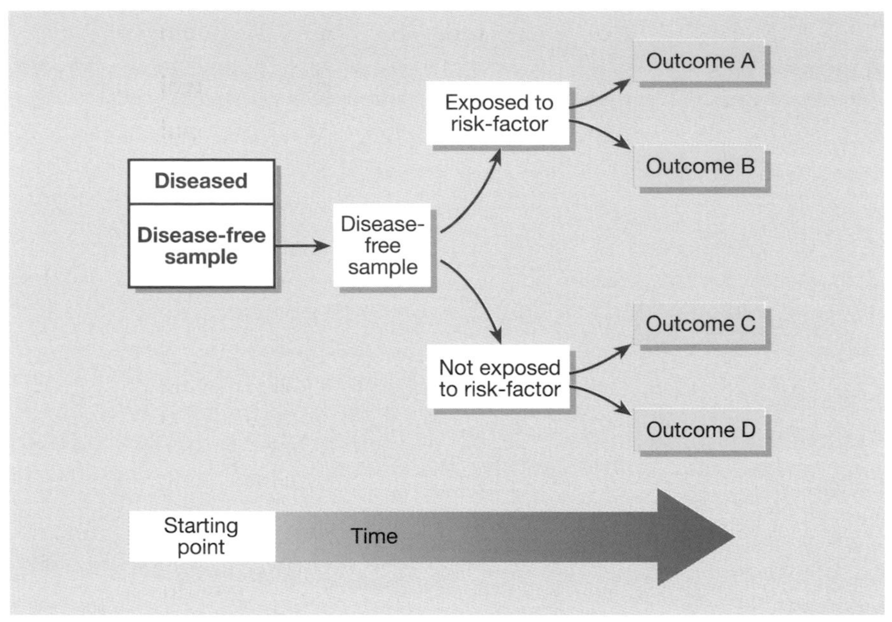

Fig 9-1 Cohort study.

The CASP Questions

Did the Study Address a Clearly Focused Issue?

As with randomised controlled trials we are looking for a clear idea of the focus of the study in terms of the population studied, any risk factors studied, the outcomes considered and clarity on whether the study tried to detect a beneficial or harmful effect.

Did the Authors Use an Appropriate Method to Answer their Question?

In other words, was a cohort study a good way of answering the question under the circumstances? Was it the right study design to choose; was a randomised controlled trial an inappropriate, unfeasible or unethical way to address the question?

Was the Cohort Recruited in an Acceptable Way?

The internal validity of a study is defined as the extent to which the observed difference in outcomes between the two comparison groups can be attributed to the intervention rather than to other factors.

Table 9-1 **Comparison of cohort studies and randomised controlled trials**

Item	Cohort studies	Randomised controlled trials
Populations studied	Diverse populations of patients who are observed in a range of settings	Highly selected populations recruited on the basis of detailed criteria and treated at selected sites
Allocation to the intervention	Based on decisions made by providers or patients	Based on chance and controlled by investigators
Outcomes	Can be defined after the intervention and can include rare or unexpected events	Primary outcomes are determined before patients are entered into study and are focused on predicted benefits and risks
Follow-up	Many cohort studies rely on existing experience (retrospective studies) and can provide an opportunity for long follow-up	Prospective studies; often have short follow-up because of costs and pressure to produce timely evidence
Analysis	Sophisticated multivariate techniques may be required to deal with confounders	Analysis is straightforward

So, we are looking to see if the study designers have tried to avoid a selection bias. Selection bias is defined by CONSORT (Altman et al., 2001) as a systematic error in creating intervention groups, causing them to differ with respect to prognosis. The groups differ in measured or unmeasured baseline characteristics because of the way in which participants were selected for the study or assigned to their study groups.

Things you need to consider are:
- Was the cohort representative of a defined population?
- Was there something special about the cohort?
- Was everybody included who should have been included?

		Yes	No	Can't tell
1.	Did the study address a clearly-focused issue?	☐	☐	☐
2.	Did the authors use an appropriate method to answer their question?	☐	☐	☐
3.	Was the cohort recruited in an acceptable way?	☐	☐	☐
4.	Was the exposure accurately measured to minimise bias?	☐	☐	☐
5.	Was the outcome accurately measured to minimise bias?	☐	☐	☐
6.	Have the authors identified all important confounding factors?	☐	☐	☐
7.	Have they taken account of the confounding factors in the design and/or analysis?	☐	☐	☐
8.	Was the follow-up of subjects complete enough?	☐	☐	☐
9.	Was the follow-up of subjects long enough?	☐	☐	☐
10.	What are the results of this study?	----------------		
11.	How precise are the results?	----------------		
12.	Do you believe the results?	☐	☐	☐
13.	Do the results of this study fit with other available evidence?	☐	☐	☐
14.	Can the results be applied to the local population?	☐	☐	☐

Fig 9-2 CASP questions to appraise a cohort study.

Was the Exposure Accurately Measured to Minimise Bias?

Here you are looking to see if there has been any bias in the way in which the exposure being studied has been measured or classified. The more objectively any given exposure can be measured the better. For example, it is well known that asking people whether or not they are still smoking may not elicit an accurate response so this is a subjective method, while measuring salivary cotinine levels is a more objective measure (van Vunakis et al., 1989).

It is also important to understand whether measures truly reflect what you are looking for and have been validated. We also need to know whether all the subjects are classified into exposure groups using the same procedures.

Have the Authors Identified All Important Confounding Factors?

Confounding is a term that describes a situation in which the estimated intervention effect is biased because of some difference between the comparison groups apart from the planned interventions. This could be baseline characteristics (e.g. socio-economic background), factors affecting prognosis (e.g. smoking status), or concurrent treatments. Age and sex are the most common confounding variables in health-related studies because these two variables are not only associated with most exposures we are interested in such as diet, smoking habits, physical exercise etc., but they are also independent risk factors for most diseases.

Which ones do you think are important and have the authors missed any important ones?

Have they Taken Account of the Confounding Factors in the Design and/or Analysis?

In a cohort study, confounding can be dealt with at the design stage of a study by:

- ***Matching***. This is normally only done for well-known confounders and selects comparison groups with similar backgrounds (e.g. non-smokers are matched with other non-smokers, while smokers are matched with other smokers).
- ***Restriction***. This limits participation in a study to specific groups that are similar to each other with respect to the confounder (e.g. if smoking is likely to be a confounder then only non-smokers will be included in the study).

Confounding can also be controlled for in the analysis by:

- ***Stratification***. Here the strength of the association is measured separately in each well-defined sub-group (e.g. regular attenders and those who attend with a problem). Using statistical techniques, overall summary measures of the association can be obtained and adjusted or controlled for the effects of the confounder.
- ***Statistical modelling***. There are more advanced techniques that simultaneously take into consideration the effects of all the possible confounders that have been recorded by the investigators.

Was the Follow-up of Subjects Complete Enough? And Was the Follow-up of Subjects Long Enough?

Cohort studies often take place over many years, with a great deal of detail being recorded for each participant. It is important that each record is as complete as possible; this may include cause of death. It is also important that loss to follow-up is as low as practical, and participants lost to follow-up may have different outcomes from those available for assessment.

The follow-up period needs to be long enough for positive or negative effects to be identified (e.g. if assessing the number of cases that progress to oral cancer in a cohort of leukoplakia patients, enough time needs to have elapsed in order to assess correctly the number of leukoplakias that transform).

In an open or dynamic cohort study where participants can enter or leave the cohort, are there any special features about the outcome of the people leaving, or the exposure of the people entering the cohort?

What Are the Results of this Study?

Ideally, as with all studies, we would like to see a clearly defined result or bottom line. We would like to see that the authors have reported the rate or the proportion between the exposed/unexposed and if absolute risk reduction and relative risks are provided.

Risk and odds

Consider this hypothetical cohort study of water fluoridation. The water in Testshire (T) had been fluoridated in February 2000. All the children born during April and May 2000 in the area had been entered into one cohort. A similar cohort from Controlshire (C) which had a very similar demographic and caries prevalence level, but was non-fluoridated, was also recruited. Detailed follow-up of all the children was undertaken looking at a range of variables. At five years of age a detailed dental examination was undertaken. In Testshire there were 1598 births during April and May 2000 and 1674 in Controlshire. At five years 1428 children were examined in Testshire and 1570 in Controlshire. Some 738 children in Controlshire were apparently free of caries (DMFT = 0) and 959 in Testshire.

If this were a real study the conclusion may well be presented as follows:

At five years of age 67.2% of children were caries-free in Testshire and 47% in Controlshire. This is clinically significant and represents an absolute risk reduction in caries at five years of age of 20%.

Cohort studies are normally analysed using a 2 × 2 table as shown in Table 9-2. If we use the data from the hypothetical study above we can see how the calculations are carried out.

Table 9-2 **2 × 2 table**

	Exposed to factor		
Disease of interest	Yes	No	Total
Yes	a	b	$a + b$
No	c	d	$c + d$
Total	$a + c$	$b + d$	$n = a + b + c + d$

Because we have followed the children over a five-year period we can estimate the risk of them getting caries.

Risk of caries =

$$\frac{\text{Number of children developing disease (caries) over period (5 years)}}{\text{Total number in cohort}}$$

$$= \frac{a + b}{n}$$

Risk of caries in the exposed (to fluoride) group =

$$R_{exp} = \frac{\text{Number of children exposed (to fluoride) with caries}}{\text{Total number exposed}}$$

$$= \frac{a}{a + c}$$

Risk of caries in the unexposed (to fluoride) group =

$$R_{unexp} = \frac{\text{Number of children exposed with caries}}{\text{Total number exposed}}$$

$$= \frac{b}{b + d}$$

The relative risk is then

$$\frac{R_{exp}}{R_{unexp}} = \frac{a / a + c}{b / b + d}$$

Relative risk (RR) is a common way of estimating the risk of experiencing a particular effect or result. If the RR equals 1 the risk is the same in both the exposed and unexposed groups. If it is larger than 1 (>1) the individual is at increased risk; if it is lower than one (<1) they are at decreased risk. For example, If the RR = 4.0, the result is about 4 times more likely to happen, and 0.25 means it is 4 times less likely to happen.

From the data given above we can fill in some of the details (Table 9-3) and calculate the rest (i.e. the number of children with caries in each group).

Table 9-3 **Completed 2 × 2 table**

	Exposed to fluoride		
Caries	Yes	No	Total
Yes	469	832	1301
No	959	738	1697
Total	1428	1570	2998

We can then calculate the results for our data:

Risk of getting caries = 1301/2998 = 0.4339

Risk of caries in the exposed (to fluoride) group (R_{exp}) = 469/1428 = 0.3284 (33%)

Risk of caries in the unexposed (to fluoride) group (R_{unexp}) = 832/1570 = 0.5299 (53%)

$$\text{Relative risk} = \frac{0.3284}{0.5299} = 0.6197$$

Other ways of expressing the treatment effect

The data also allow us to express the treatment effect in other ways. While the risk of getting caries in the fluoride group is 0.33 or 33%, the risk (chance) of not getting caries in the exposed (to fluoride) group is

= 1 − 0.33 = 0.67 (67%)

Similarly, the risk of caries in the unexposed group = 0.53 (53%) and the chance of not getting caries in the unexposed (to fluoride) group = 1 – 0.53 = 0.47 (47%).

We can also calculate absolute risk reduction (ARR), relative risk reduction, and numbers needed to treat as before (see pages 54 and 72).

Absolute risk reduction. The difference in risk between the two groups

= Risk in exposed fluoride group – Risk in unexposed group

= 67% – 47%

= 20%

The ***relative risk reduction***

$$= \frac{\text{Risk in exposed fluoride group} - \text{Risk in unexposed group}}{\text{Risk in unexposed group}}$$

$$= \frac{67\% - 47\%}{47\%}$$

= 42.6% (43%)

The ***number needed to treat*** (NNT)

$$= \frac{100}{\text{Absolute risk reduction}}$$ for percentages (or 1/ARR)

$$= \frac{100}{20}$$

= 5

So using the same set of data from our hypothetical study, summarised in Table 9-3, we have outlined how to calculate some common methods of expressing a study's results. Some of these measures are summarised in Table 9-4. If you were a salesperson trying to promote this intervention, which of these would you choose?

Table 9-4 **Summary of measures**

Chance of not getting caries in the fluoridated group	67%
Absolute risk reduction	20%
Relative risk reduction	43%
Numbers needed to treat	5

The important point here is that you appreciate that they are all relatively simple to derive and they are all come from the same data.

Odds ratios

Relative risks are relatively well understood by patients and clinicians. However, odds ratios have appealing mathematical properties and are frequently used in systematic reviews so it is useful to understand how they are calculated. Odds ratios are also commonly used in case–controlled studies to measure the association between exposure and risk of disease. Indeed, Deeks (1998) has argued that they should only be used in case–controlled studies and logistic regression analyses.

Because they are also used on occasion as a measure of effect size in cohort studies, the same data as above can be used to illustrate how to calculate odds ratios.

$$\text{Odds of being a case (having caries) in exposed group} = \frac{a}{c} = \frac{469}{959} = 0.4890$$

$$\text{Odds of being a case (having caries) in unexposed group} = \frac{b}{d} = \frac{832}{738} = 1.1274$$

$$\text{Odds ratio} = \frac{\text{Odds of being a case (having caries) in exposed group}}{\text{Odds of being a case (having caries) in unexposed group}}$$

$$= \frac{0.4890}{1.1274}$$

$$= 0.4338$$

How Precise Are the Results?

As explained on page 72, the precision of the study can be measured by the size of the confidence intervals (CIs). The narrower the CI, the more precise the estimate of the effect of the treatment under investigation.

The risk ratio diagram

In the risk ratio diagram (Fig 9-3) it can be seen that the mean value of the result is represented as a circle (or square). The size of this circle is sometimes used to represent the sample size, being bigger with large samples. The horizontal lines represent the size of the confidence intervals, so the longer the confidence intervals the less precise the result. If the confidence intervals cross the line of no effect (i.e. the 95% confidence intervals include 1), the result is not significant.

For a result to be significant, the mean value of a study and its confidence intervals must lie wholly one side or other of the line of no effect. Which side of the line depends on the outcome of interest.

This type of diagram is often used to summarise the results in systematic reviews. It enables you to assess very rapidly the overall picture, and see the

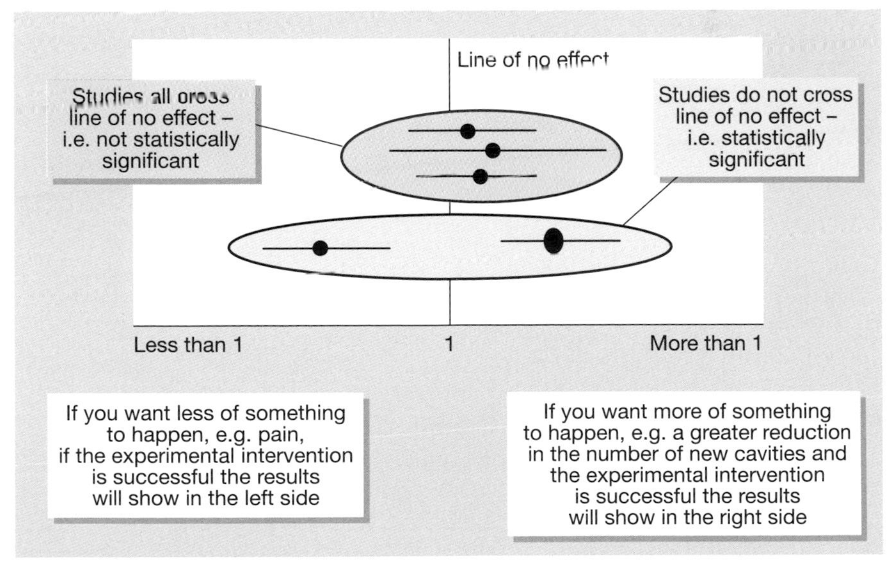

Fig 9-3 Risk ratio diagram.

wood from the trees; hence it is also called a forest plot (Fig 9-4) or more colloquially a "blobbogram".

Analysis 01.03. Comparison 01 Fluoride Varnish versus Placebo/No-treatment, Outcome 03 D(M)FS increment (SMD) - nearest to 3 years (7 trials)

Review: Fluoride varnishes for preventing dental caries in children and adolescents
Comparison: 01 Fluoride Varnish versus Placebo/No-treatment
Outcome: 03 D(M)FS increment (SMD) - nearest to 3 years (7 trials)

Study	Fluoride Varnish N	Fluoride Varnish Mean(SD)	Placebo/NT N	Placebo/NT Mean(SD)	Standardised Mean Difference (Random) 95% CI	Weight (%)	Standardised Mean Difference (Random) 95% CI
Borutta 1991	270	2.07 (2.34)	90	2.90 (3.60)		15.3	-0.31 [-0.55, -0.07]
Bravo 1997	98	1.48 (2.20)	116	2.58 (2.63)		14.3	-0.45 [-0.72, -0.18]
Clark 1985	442	2.50 (3.14)	234	3.11 (3.54)		17.5	-0.19 [-0.34, -0.03]
Koch 1975	60	0.90 (3.80)	61	4.00 (3.75)		11.5	-0.82 [-1.19, -0.44]
Modeer 1984	87	1.40 (2.28)	107	2.00 (2.78)		14.0	-0.23 [-0.52, 0.05]
Tewari 1990	311	0.55 (4.59)	307	2.16 (4.03)		17.5	-0.37 [-0.53, -0.21]
Holm 1984	42	1.43 (1.50)	53	3.15 (1.31)		9.8	-1.22 [-1.66, -0.78]
Total (95% CI)	1310		968			100.0	-0.46 [-0.65, -0.26]

Test for heterogeneity chi-square=26.41 df=6 p=0.0002 I^2 =77.3%
Test for overall effect z=4.57 p<0.00001

-4.0 -2.0 0 2.0 4.0
Favours F varnish Favours placebo/NT

Fig 9-4 Example of forest plot from a systematic review. (Marinho VCC, Higgins JPT, Logan S, Sheiham A. Fluoride varnishes for preventing dental caries in children and adolescents. *Cochrane Database of Systematic Reviews* 2002, Issue 1. Art. No.: CD002279).

Do You Believe the Results?

After identifying the study's bottom line and the precision of results, you need to ask yourself if you believe the results. A big effect is hard to ignore but you need to be sure that it is not due to any biases, chance or confounding. You also need to be sure that the study methodology is robust enough to rely on the results.

Association and causation

Another important issue is to distinguish between cause and association. Simply because two factors or conditions are associated, it does not necessarily follow that one is the cause of the other.

For example, in a developing new town, figures indicate that the number of dentists are increasing and the consumption of alcohol is increasing in proportion to the number of dentists. It could be said that the increase in the number of dentists is associated with the increasing alcohol consumption.

This does not mean that the dentists are drinking all the alcohol! It is much more likely that the increase in population of the new town has resulted in the increased alcohol consumption and that dentists have been attracted to the area by the same increase in population.

In 1965 Bradford Hill (see Hill, 1965) proposed a number of aspects to be considered to help judge whether an observed effect was causal.

Time sequence. The exposure must precede the outcome (although measurement of the exposure is not required to precede measurement of the outcome).

Dose–response gradient. The likelihood of a causal association is increased if a biological gradient or dose–response curve can be demonstrated (e.g. heavier smokers are at greater risk of lung cancer).

Strength. Bradford Hill suggested that strong associations were more likely to be causal than weak associations. The strong associations he cites (a 200-fold increase in mortality from scrotal cancer in chimney sweeps exposed to tar or mineral oils, and a 20-fold increased risk of lung cancer in smokers compared with non-smokers) have more credence, being less likely to be attributable solely to uncontrolled residual confounding. Relatively weak associations are common in contemporary epidemiology.

Plausibility. While it is reassuring if a causal association is biologically plausible, Bradford Hill notes that *"this is a feature I am convinced we cannot demand. What is biologically plausible depends upon the biological knowledge of the day"*. Further, it is *"too often based not on logic or data but only on prior beliefs"*.

Consistency. Bradford Hill also felt more confidence in a causal explanation for an association if the same answer had been achieved in a variety of different situations – prospectively and retrospectively and in different populations.

Specificity. This criterion is often stated to mean that any exposure may give rise to only a single outcome. While this may be true for some infectious diseases – for example, only rubella virus causes rubella – it is clearly unlikely with respect to many environmental exposures. Bradford Hill recognised that diseases may have more than one cause and that one-to-one relationships are not frequent. However, if an association is limited to specific groups with a particular environmental exposure or is greatly increased in these groups, then the case for a causal association is strengthened. Weiss (2002) suggests resurrection of specificity as a useful concept in study design, particularly valuable in unravelling complex problems in causal attribution.

Coherence. Coherence and biological plausibility share a requirement that the cause-and-effect interpretation of an association should fit with the known facts of the natural history and biology of the disease.

Experiment. Do preventive actions taken on the basis of a demonstrated cause-and-effect association alter the frequency of the outcome? With overtones of Koch's postulates, this criterion offered, in Bradford Hill's view, the strongest support of a causal interpretation.

Do the Results of this Study Fit with Other Available Evidence?

This highlights one of Bradford Hill's criteria of consistency of evidence.

Can the Results be Applied to the Local Population?

The application of the results to the local population or your own patients is always the key question and you need to consider whether:

- The subjects covered in the study could be sufficiently different from your population to cause concern.
- Your local setting is likely to differ much from that of the study.

Key Points

- Well-designed and executed cohort studies are important to defining the evidence-base. They can help provide answers when randomised controlled trials are inappropriate or impossible to conduct.
- A simple 10-question tool for the appraisal of cohort studies has been outlined. This is available from www.phru.nhs.uk/Pages/PHD/resources.htm.
- Risk and odds ratios and association/causations are explained.

References

Altman DG, Schulz KF, Moher D, Egger M, Davidoff F, Elbourne D et al. The revised CONSORT statement for reporting randomized trials: explanation and elaboration. Ann Intern Med 2001;134:663–694. (www.consort-statement.org).

Black N. Why we need observational studies to evaluate the effectiveness of health care. Br Med J 1996;312(7040):1215–1218.

Deeks J. When can odds ratios mislead? Br Med J 1998;317(7166):1155.

Hill AB. The environment and disease: association or causation? Proc R Soc Med 1965;58:295–300.

van Vunakis H, Tashkin DP, Rigas B, Simmons M, Gjika HB, Clark VA. Relative sensitivity and specificity of salivary and serum cotinine in identifying tobacco-smoking status of self-reported nonsmokers and smokers of tobacco and/or marijuana. Arch Environ Health 1989;44(1):53–58.

Weiss NS. Can the "specificity" of an association be rehabilitated as a basis for supporting a causal hypothesis? Epidemiology 2002;13:6–8.

Additional Reading

Lucas RM, McMichael AJ. Association or causation: evaluating links between "environment and disease". Bull World Health Org 2005;83(10):792–795. Epub 2005 Nov 10.

Mamdani M, Sykora K, Li P, Normand SL, Streiner DL, Austin PC et al. Reader's guide to critical appraisal of cohort studies: 2. Assessing potential for confounding. Br Med J 2005;330(7497):960–962.

Mann CJ. Observational research methods. Research design II: cohort, cross sectional, and case–control studies. Emerg Med J 2003;20(1):54–60.

Normand SL, Sykora K, Li P, Mamdani M, Rochon PA, Anderson GM. Reader's guide to critical appraisal of cohort studies: 3. Analytical strategies to reduce confounding. Br Med J 2005;330(7498):1021–1023.

Rochon PA, Gurwitz JH, Sykora K, Mamdani M, Streiner DL, Garfinkel S et al. Reader's guide to critical appraisal of cohort studies: 1. Role and design. Br Med J 2005;330(7496):895–897.

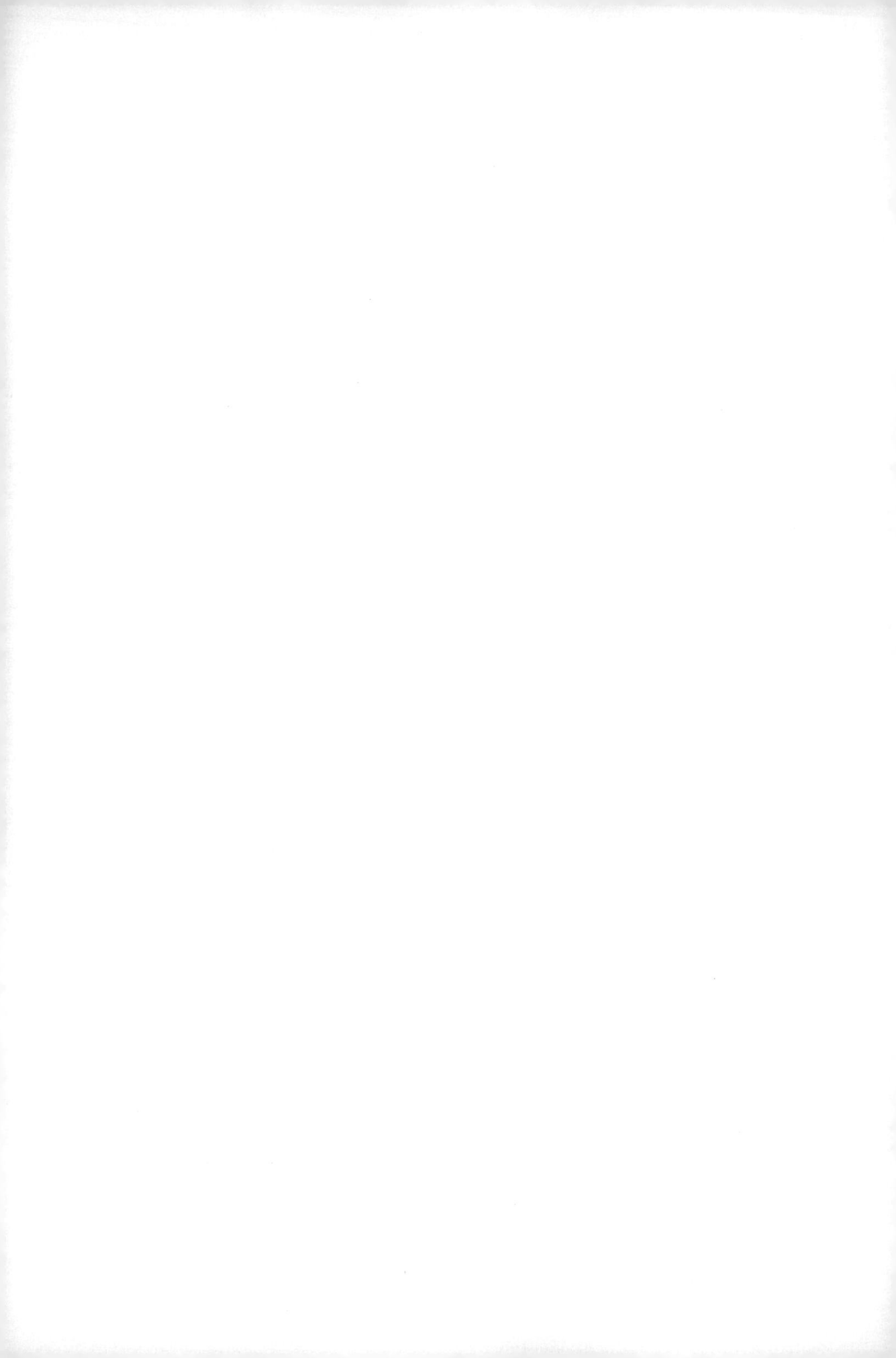

Chapter 10

Study Appraisal: Diagnostic Studies

Aim

The aim of this chapter is to outline how to appraise a diagnostic study using measures such as sensitivity and specificity to determine the effectiveness of tests.

Outcomes

After completing this chapter readers should be able to appraise a diagnostic study, understand and be able to calculate sensitivity, specificity, negative and positive predictive values and likelihood ratios.

What are Diagnostic Tests?

Unlike the introduction of new treatments, there are very few barriers to the introduction of new diagnostic tests, as these are judged by using somewhat less stringent criteria than, for example, drugs. As a result, new diagnostic tests are constantly being developed and marketed.

A diagnostic test or investigation can be used for a variety of purposes. It can diagnose a condition, help assess the severity of a disease, predict the prognosis of a disease, monitor changes or responses to treatment, or be used for screening, risk assessment or to establish baseline values.

It should be noted that when screening is discussed it is normally in relation to a single test. However, screening actually consists of all the stages in a programme for identification of the individual at risk. While most people are aware of the Wilson and Jungner criteria for screening (see Wilson and Jungner, 1968), the UK National Screening committee has developed criteria for screening programmes more relevant to the evidence-based era. These relate to the condition itself, the screening test(s) and treatment available, and the screening programme. These criteria are available at the specialist screening library (www.library.nhs.uk/screening).

With an increasing number of diagnostic tests being made available it is important to be able to appraise the quality of the studies supporting these tests. As with systematic reviews and randomised controlled trials, CASP has developed a tool (Fig 10-1) to help appraise diagnostic tests (based on a paper by Jaesche et al., 1994).

The CASP Questions

Was There a Clear Question for the Study to Address?

The first question, as always, is whether the researchers are clear about what they are trying to do. Here we can look at the population, the test, the setting in which it is being performed and the outcomes being measured.

Was There a Comparison with an Appropriate Reference Standard?

If we were looking at a new machine for diagnosing caries, for example, we would ideally want to compare it against a robust reference standard such as

	Yes	No	Can't tell
1. Was there a clear question for the study to address?	☐	☐	☐
2. Was there a comparison with an appropriate reference standard?	☐	☐	☐
3. Did all patients get the diagnostic test and the reference standard?	☐	☐	☐
4. Could the results of the test of interest have been influenced by the results of the reference standard?	☐	☐	☐
5. Is the disease status of the tested population clearly described?	☐	☐	☐
6. Were the methods for performing the test described in sufficient detail?	☐	☐	☐
7. What are the results?	----------------		
8. How sure are we about these results?	----------------		
9. Can the results be applied to your patients/the population of interest?	☐	☐	☐
10. Can the test be applied to your patient or population of interest?	☐	☐	☐
11. Were all outcomes important to the individual or population considered?	☐	☐	☐
12. What would be the impact of using this test on your patients/population?	----------------		

Fig 10-1 CASP appraisal questions for diagnostic tests.

histological confirmation or direct visual examination. While dental radiographs are a useful adjunct, they have a number of limitations when used alone to diagnose caries.

Did All Patients Get the Diagnostic Test and the Reference Standard?

It is important that all patients receive both the test under evaluation and the reference, or gold standard, test. This is because diagnostic tests are never 100% accurate. There are always people who test positive even though they don't have the disease/condition (false positives), and people who test negative when they do have the disease/condition under consideration (false negatives).

Could the Results of the Test of Interest have been Influenced by the Results of the Reference Standard?

When conducting the test it is important that those carrying out the test are unaware of the results of the reference standard. This can be achieved by the use of "blinding" of the examiner, or having the reference test and the new test performed independently. What we are trying to avoid is a *review bias*.

Is the Disease Status of the Tested Population Clearly Described?

It is important to know the presenting symptoms, disease stage or severity of the condition under test as well as any co-morbidities and potential differential diagnoses. This gives us a clear picture of the conditions in which the test is effective or not. We need to know at what stage of the disease or condition the test is most effective. For example, a new caries diagnostic test may be tested on only those teeth with obvious clinical signs of the disease. It might then be used to diagnose caries at an earlier stage in the disease process when the test is effective only in later stages of the disease; in this instance it may fail to detect caries that is really there. Consequently, it is important that the test is evaluated across a wide spectrum of the disease or condition to ensure appropriate use in the future. This controls for *spectrum bias*.

Were the Methods for Performing the Test Described in Sufficient Detail?

Sufficient details about how the test was conducted should be provided in the study in order for us to carry out the test ourselves, if necessary.

How Sure are You About These Results?

If you are happy with the findings after answering the above questions, it is worth looking at the results in detail. If not, you can ignore them and look for another paper.

To determine how well a test performs we need to be able to calculate the sensitivity and specificity of the test.

Sensitivity is also known as the true positive rate. In other words, it is the probability that a patient with the disease will test positive (detection rate).

Specificity tells us how good the test is at excluding people without the condition, or the true negative rate. It is defined as the probability that a patient who is disease-free will have a negative test result.

In a good study, values for sensitivity and specificity of the test should be provided, but if not they can be calculated easily using a 2 × 2 table (Table 10-1) if the information is provided.

Table 10-1 **Calculating diagnostic test measures**

	Reference standard		
	Disease present	Disease absent	
Test positive	a	b	$a + b$
Test negative	c	d	$c + d$
Total	$a + c$	$b + d$	$a + b + c + d$

a = true positive; those with the disease or condition who test positive for it with the new test.
b = false positive; those without the disease who test positive with the new test (i.e. the test incorrectly identifies this group as needing treatment).
c = false negative; those who have the condition or disease, but test negative (and thus not getting the treatment they need).
d = true negative; those without the disease who (correctly) test negative for the disease.

Sensitivity (detection rate) $= \dfrac{\text{All those with the disease who test positive}}{\text{All those with the disease}}$

$$= \frac{a}{a + c}$$

$$\text{Specificity} = \frac{\text{All those who test negative who don't have the disease}}{\text{All those without the disease}}$$

$$= \frac{d}{b + d}$$

Ideally, both sensitivity and specificity should be high (close to 100%). Because of the way tests work, it is more likely that sensitivity is sacrificed for specificity and vice versa. The ramifications of finding all the diseased patients, or not missing any healthy patients, help to decide which property is more important. For example, in a disease with high mortality or morbidity, you want a test with high sensitivity. This means few cases are missed. High specificity is useful for screening tests, and when the *treatment* for the condition has high morbidity. This means fewer healthy people are subjected to unnecessary treatment.

Sensitivity and specificity provide information about the performance of the test, but what do these properties mean to the patient? We can calculate the chance that if you test positive you have the disease, and the chance that if you have a negative test you don't have the disease using the same 2 × 2 table as before.

Positive predictive value. This is the probability of those testing/screening positive actually having the disease (the chance that if you test positive you have the disease).

Negative predictive value. This is the probability of those testing/screening negative *not* actually having the disease (the chance that if you have a negative test you don't have the disease).

$$\text{Positive predictive value} = \frac{\text{All those with the disease who test positive}}{\text{All those with a positive test}}$$

$$= \frac{a}{a + b}$$

$$\text{Negative predictive value} = \frac{\text{All those without the disease who test negative}}{\text{All those with a negative test}}$$

$$= \frac{d}{c + d}$$

The major problem with predictive values is they are entirely dependent upon the prevalence of the disease in the sample being tested and can therefore vary in different populations.

Likelihood ratios

When assessing the effectiveness of a test, some people find dealing with sensitivity and specificity difficult. An alternative is to use likelihood ratios. Likelihood ratios express the results of a test in terms of the chance that a person has the condition if the test reaches a given level, rather than just "diseased" or "healthy".

The likelihood ratio (LR) can be calculated from the sensitivity and specificity of a test, and is expressed as a ratio rather than a percentage. It expresses the odds that a given finding would occur in a patient with, as opposed to without, the target disorder or condition. It is derived as:

$$LR = \frac{\text{Sensitivity}}{(1 - \text{Specificity})}$$

With the LR above 1, the probability of the disease or condition being present goes up; when it is below 1 the probability of it being present goes down, and when it is exactly 1 the probability is unchanged.

Exercise

As an exercise, calculate the sensitivity, specificity, positive and negative predictive values and likelihood ratio from the following data (Table 10-2). Answers on page 128.

Table 10-2 **Data to calculate sensitivity, specificity, positive and negative predictive values and likelihood ratio**

	Reference standard		
	Disease present	Disease absent	
Test positive	215	16	231
Test negative	15	114	129
Total	230	130	360

Will the Results Help Me and My Patients/Population?
New tests are being introduced all the time and as an individual practitioner you are likely to be more concerned about whether the results of a test are important for your individual patients. However, if you manage or advise a large practice or number of practices or health services you will be more interested in the potential impact that the test could have on the population you serve.

Can the Results be Applied to Your Patients/the Population of Interest?
It is sometimes better to think of this question from the other perspective and think "are my patients/population so different from those in the study that the results cannot be applied?"

Can the Test be Applied to Your Patient or Population of Interest?
If the results of the test could be applied to your patients/population you then need to consider whether it is possible to use the test. However, there may be other considerations besides whether the test would work. It may require additional resources to use it, equipment, staff training (in the practice or laboratory) and additional laboratory costs. There may also be an impact on the way that you currently provide services.

Were All Outcomes Important to the Individual or Population Considered?
There are often outcomes that have not been considered, and you need to decide from your perspective whether the studies have omitted to consider any outcomes that are relevant to your individual patients or population.

What Would be the Impact of Using this Test on Your Patients/Population?
Again you need to consider any impact relevant to your practice population, be it one patient or thousands.

Key Points

- New diagnostic tests are being developed with increasing frequency. You need to be able to decide whether these tests will help you and your patients.
- A simple 10-question tool, available for the appraisal of diagnostic studies, is outlined. This is available from: www.phru.nhs.uk/Pages/PHD/resources.htm.

References

Jaesche R, Guyatt GH, Sackett DL. Users' guides to the medical literature, VI. How to use an article about a diagnostic test. J Am Med Assoc 1994;271(5):389–391.

Wilson JMG, Jungner G. Principles and Practice of Screening for Disease. Public Health Paper No. 34. Geneva: World Health Organization, 1968.

Additional Reading

Bossuyt, PM et al. Towards complete and accurate reporting of studies of diagnostic accuracy: The STARD initiative, Jan. 2003. See www.consort-statement.org/stardstatement.htm.

Deeks JJ. Systematic reviews in health care: systematic reviews of evaluations of diagnostic and screening tests. Br Med J 2001;323:157–162.

Greenhalgh T. How to read a paper: Papers that report diagnostic or screening tests. Br Med J 1997;315:540–543.

Loong T-W. Understanding sensitivity and specificity with the right side of the brain. Br Med J 2003;327:716–719.

Moher D, Cook DJ, Eastwood S, Olkin I, Rennie D, Stroup DF. Improving the quality of reports of meta-analyses of randomised controlled trials: the QUOROM statement. Quality of reporting of meta-analyses. Lancet 1999;354:1896–1900.

Whiting P, Rutjes AW, Dinnes J, Reitsma J, Bossuyt PM, Kleijnen J. Development and validation of methods for assessing the quality of diagnostic accuracy studies. Health Technol Assess 2004;8(25):1–234.

Whiting P, Rutjes AW, Reitsma JB, Bossuyt PM, Kleijnen J. The development of QUADAS: a tool for the quality assessment of studies of diagnostic accuracy included in systematic reviews. BMC Med Res Methodol 2003;3:25.

Whiting P, Rutjes AW, Reitsma JB, Glas AS, Bossuyt PM, Kleijnen J. Sources of variation and bias in studies of diagnostic accuracy: a systematic review. Ann Intern Med 2004;140(3):189–202.

Chapter 11

Study Appraisal: Qualitative Studies

Aim

The aim of this chapter is to provide an overview of qualitative research and its appraisal.

Outcomes

After completing this chapter readers will be aware of the range of qualitative research and be aware of the questions that need to be addressed in appraising qualitative research.

What is Qualitative Research?

Qualitative research looks at people's experiences, attitudes and beliefs or their perceptions of a situation. In healthcare it has been used to help generate new theories, understand patients' and clinicians' behaviour, to develop appropriate interventions, evaluate healthcare policy or systems of care and to enhance and help explain quantitative data.

Qualitative research can be used to address such issues as what it is like to live with a certain condition (e.g trigeminal neuralgia) or what it is like to have a diagnosis of oral cancer.

Qualitative methods include techniques such as interviews, focus groups, observation and a wide range of approaches. They could include the following:

- ***Phenomenology***. This looks at how people see their world.
- ***Grounded theory***. This method emanates from sociology and aims to generate theory from data using a range of techniques noted above.
- ***Ethnography***. This approach is developed from anthropology and looks at behaviour within a culture
- ***Critical theory***. Here the approach is to specifically increase people's understanding of their situation and through this they initiate change.

In general, qualitative research attempts to understand human action through a collection of individual accounts of subjective experiences. It adopts an "inductive approach" where knowledge is generated rather than tested, as in the quantitative approach where a hypothetico-deductive approach is taken, seeking to explain behaviour through the verification and falsification of hypotheses.

Black (1994) argued for the value of qualitative research in healthcare research and later Sackett and Wennberg (1997) emphasised that it was the research question itself that should be the determining factor in research design.

It is clear that high-quality qualitative and quantitative research is necessary to improve the effectiveness of healthcare delivery. Consequently there is a need for appraisal of qualitative literature as there is in the quantitative literature. Popay et al. (1998) provide a useful framework but they argue that there is no absolute list or criteria, and Mays and Pope (2000) highlight the fact that there are no easy solutions to limit the likelihood that there will be errors in qualitative research.

However, some guidance can be given in what to look for when appraising qualitative research, and key elements to consider in good qualitative research are:
- clarity
- validity
- theoretical adequacy
- generalisability.

Clarity
In our appraisal of quantitative research we are looking for a clearly defined research question where the population, intervention and outcomes were likely to be indicated at the outset. The nature of qualitative research means that outcomes are seldom if ever known at the outset. Consequently what we need to see in the research is clarity about what researchers are trying to accomplish.

Validity
In terms of assessing validity there are a number of questions that can be considered:
- Did the study measure what it set out to measure?
- Has an appropriate sample been selected?
- Can the data be verified?
- Are the findings reliable?
- Are the findings relevant to the original question?

Did the study measure what it set out to measure?
In quantitative research this is known as internal validity; in qualitative research it is termed credibility. You are looking to see whether the researchers have accessed and accurately represented the social world under study.

Has an appropriate sample been selected?
Sampling in qualitative research is usually purposeful, so you are looking to see if the sample has been selected in such a manner that the researchers are likely to get the information they are looking for. This requires a clear description of the way in which sampling was undertaken.

Can the data be verified?
Triangulation is one method of verifying data where the results of one or more methods of data collection are compared (e.g. interviews and observation). The findings can also be fed back to participants, which is called respondent validation or verification.

Are the findings reliable?
An issue to consider here is whether the findings accurately reflect features of the phenomena under discussion. This is easiest to do if the findings are coherently presented, with some assurance that the material was accurately checked. The researcher should move from describing the data, through quotation or examples, to analysis or interpretation of the meaning and significance. You need to assess whether the account was fair and balanced and took into account multiple perspectives, interests and realities (completeness).

Theoretical adequacy
It is recognised that the researcher's perceptions and background have an influence on the questions asked, the data obtained, and their interpretation in qualitative research. (In reality these are often present in quantitative research as well.) What is important is whether the findings are plausible or have explanatory power.

Things to look out for are whether the researcher articulates the relationship between the data and the original theoretical argument in a clear fashion, and whether links between the data and comments on what the data contain are made. Also, is evidence both for and against the argument being made or the theory being postulated presented, and are paradoxes, contradictions or inconsistencies in the data explained?

The researcher should present the data and theoretical discussion together in such a way as to "make sense" of what is known from other studies and discuss whether the findings are generalisable (transferable) to other bodies of knowledge or populations/groups.

Generalisability
In quantitative research generalisability is sometimes referred to as external validity. In qualitative research it is referred to as fittingness – that is, whether the findings are applicable to people and situations that are similar to the ones that were researched.

Unlike in quantitative research, where samples are chosen to be representative so that the results can be generalised, in qualitative research the participants are usually selected because they possess specific characteristics the researcher is interested in addressing. So what you need to look for in qualitative research is whether the researcher describes explicitly the context in which the study takes place.

The description should be good enough to allow you to decide whether your patients are similar to those in the study so that you can decide whether the recommendations are appropriate and acceptable in your context and therefore relevant for your patients.

Key Points

- High-quality qualitative research is as necessary as high-quality quantitative research to improve the effectiveness of healthcare.
- Tools for appraising qualitative research do exist and are being further developed. However, there are no easy solutions to limit the likelihood that there will be errors in qualitative research.

References

Black N. Why we need qualitative research. J Epidemiol Community Health 1994;48(5):425–426.

Mays N, Pope C. Qualitative research in health care. Assessing quality in qualitative research. Br Med J 2000;320(7226):50–52.

Popay J, Rogers A, Williams G. Rationale and standards for the systematic review of qualitative literature in health services research. Qual Health Res 1998;8(3):341–351.

Sackett DL, Wennberg JE. Choosing the best research design for each question. Br Med J 1997;315(7123):1636.

Additional Reading

Greenhalgh T, Taylor R. Papers that go beyond numbers (qualitative research). Br Med J 1997;315(7110):740–743.

Mays N, Pope C (eds). Qualitative research in health care. London: BMJ Books, 1999.

Seers K. Qualitative Research. In: Evidence-based Primer for Health Care Professionals. Dawes et al. (eds). Edinburgh: Churchill Livingstone, 1999:111–126

Chapter 12

Keeping Up To Date

Aim

The aim of this chapter is to outline a number of strategies to help your practice become more evidence-based.

Outcomes

After completing this chapter you will be aware of a number of strategies that will assist you in practising in an evidence-based manner.

Applying and Evaluating the Best Available Evidence

In this book we have attempted to illustrate a practical approach to evidence-based practice. This has been based on the 5 As of the evidence-based approach (Table 12-1).

While this text can help you develop the first three elements, the final two need definite action on your part. This is because it is the application of the best available evidence in practice that will bring benefits to you and your patients.

Develop an Inquiring Mind

Evidence-based practice is all about asking questions, so develop an enquiring mind. Healthcare professionals, as a whole, tend to be patriarchal. Consciously

Table 12-1 **The evidence-based method**

ASK	Asking answerable questions
ACQUIRE	Searching for the best evidence
APPRAISE	Critically appraising the evidence
APPLY	Applying the evidence
ASSESS	Evaluating the outcome

or not, we advocate a plan for a patient or a belief about a condition rather than enquire into the best possible approach. For example, most of us will say "I think ...", "I believe ...", "The facts are ...", "Experience says ...", and "My colleagues always ...". Enquiry, on the other hand, is characterised by such statements as: "I wonder whether there is a better way?", "Should I keep doing this?" and "Why have I always ...?". When you find yourself making advocacy statements, you may wish to question what you thought was "true". While advocacy tends to uphold the status quo, enquiry leads to new knowledge and new insights. It keeps you up to date and patients appreciate the fact that you are making the effort to do so.

Educational Prescriptions

When you have these thoughts or encounter a clinical problem, write them down and convert them into a PICO question and write yourself an educational prescription (www.cebm.net/index.aspx?o=1036). Instead of reading that latest freebie dental magazine, spend some time searching on the internet to see if you can find the information to answer the question you have set yourself.

Critically Appraised Topics

If you do find a paper and appraise it to answer your question, you might want to write it down formally as a short critically appraised topic (CAT) for your own use. For more details of how to do this and some free software to assist, visit the Centre for Evidence-Based Medicine's CAT page at www.cebm.net/index.aspx?o=1157.

Practise, Practise, Practise

Like learning how to cut your first cavity preparation or scale subgingivally, practising in an evidence-based manner means doing it again and again until it becomes second nature. Become an effective computer user. It takes practice but will save you time in the long run. Many dentists now have computers in their offices. Excellent sources of evidence-based information for desktop computers can be found at the Centre for Evidence-based Dentistry (CEBD) at www.cebd.org.

Developing your appraisal skills also takes time; you could do this with a group of colleagues locally, attend a course or make use of some of the online materials available. There are some links at the CEBD at www.cebd.org/?o=1053.

Identify Useful Resources

We have suggested the following hierarchy for you to follow to find information to answer clinical problems:

Evidence-based **G**uidelines
Cochrane reviews
Systematic reviews
Studies

One way to remember this is with the mnemonic: **G**ood **C**linicians **S**eek **S**cience.

However, there is a range of resources that seek to synthesise and summarise the available good-quality evidence to help speed up the process. Two of these are paper-based journals:

- *The Evidence-based Dentistry Journal*
- *The Journal of Evidence-based Dental Practice.*

You then have three websites:

- the Oral Health Specialist library (www.library.nhs.uk/oralhealth)
- the Centre for Evidence-based Dentistry (www.cebd.org)
- the Pan American Centers for Evidence Based Dentistry (www.evidentista.org).

These three resources are continuing to develop and while the sites are all slightly different, at their core they all provide a range of summarised evidence-based information (see Chapter 13 for more details).

Apply the Best Available Evidence in Clinical Practice

Knowing what to do and how to do it is one thing; however, perhaps the most difficult thing is then to apply it in practice. Most of the evidence that we have about implementing change in practice comes from the medical sector (Bero et al., 1998) and this tends to be about implementing guidelines and other more significant changes (Table 12-2). However, in your own practice with your own patients it is potentially easier for you to make changes.

Evaluate the Outcomes of Changes You Make

If you do make changes you could audit them to see if they do indeed make a difference. There is currently a trend to move research into practice which may present opportunities for you to not only develop your own evidence-based practice but also to influence others.

Table 12-2 **Interventions to improve implementation**

	Consistently effective interventions	**Interventions of variable effectiveness**	**Interventions that have little or no effect**
Educational outreach visits	✓		
Reminders (manual or computerised)	✓		
Multifaceted interventions (a combination that includes two or more of: audit and feedback, reminders, local consensus processes, or marketing)	✓		
Interactive educational meetings (workshops that include discussion or practice)	✓		
Audit and feedback		✓	
The use of local opinion leaders		✓	
Local consensus processes		✓	
Patient mediated interventions		✓	
Educational materials (e.g. clinical practice guidelines, audiovisual materials, and electronic publications)			✓
Didactic educational meetings (such as lectures)			✓

Reference

Bero L et al. Closing the gap between research and practice: an overview of systematic reviews of interventions to promote the implementation of research findings. Br Med J 1998;317:465–468.

Chapter 13

Sources of Evidence/Information

Aim

The aim of this chapter is to briefly outline some of the major sources of information available.

Outcomes

After completing this chapter you will be aware of a range of databases and other electronic resources to obtain information.

Traditional

Traditionally, dentists, like other healthcare professionals, have found their evidence from:

- lectures
- books
- journals.

Lectures/Seminars

For those with academic links or who are regular attendees at postgraduate meetings, a lecture by an expert is often a useful way of keeping in touch. However, the traditional lecture has been shown to be of little use for postgraduate education apart from the imparting of facts, much of which (75%) will be forgotten. Your own notes (if they can be read) may provide you with sources for future study, while the speaker may provide handouts with references which could be useful later. Most lectures however, although of interest, are rarely of immediate clinical importance to you or your patients and as such will be rapidly forgotten.

Books

Textbooks are a source of reference for many. However, they date rapidly and due to the publishing process many are out of date as soon as, if not before, they are published.

Journals

There are an increasing number of journals being published in the biomedical field – reputedly over 30,000 worldwide. Of these, in excess of 500 are specific to dentistry alone, with some 400 of these being referenced on MEDLINE, the bibliographic database (see later). Journals come in all shapes and sizes, from the highly esoteric single-issue variety such as *Caries Research*, through to general journals such as the *British Dental Journal*. The quality control or peer review processes varies from the strict to the non-existent.

These journals present a vast array of information to the practising dentist, not all of which is good quality or readily available. For example, research in three specialities has given some indication of how many articles in a wide range of journals a dentist in these specialities would need to read per week to keep up to date (Table 13-1).

Table 13-1 **How much do you need to read to keep up to date?**

	Articles per week	No. of journals
Paedodontics[1]	24	75
Prosthetics[2]	8	60
Endodontics[3]	3	120

[1]Yang et al., 2001; [2]Nishimura et al., 2002; [3]Kim et al., 2001.

Papers in journals are often published a year or two following the data collection and in one example in a new journal the data presented related to material more than 20 years old, which was not immediately obvious to the reader.

Modern

The coming of the information age, with the development of the internet, the move to electronic publishing and changes in printing technology, has led to a major increase in the amount of scientific literature.

The development of PubMed, a freely accessible database providing access to citations from the biomedical literature, by the National Center for Biotechnology Information (NCBI) at the National Library of Medicine (NLM), located at the US National Institutes of Health (NIH) in the USA, and the National Electronic Library for Health (now the National Library for Health) in the UK, were highly significant in this regard.

The evidence-based movement has seen the development of secondary journals in a range of areas – medicine, mental health, dentistry. These journals all produce short summaries of high-quality evidence, significantly reducing the number of articles that practitioners need to keep up to date. In addition the internet has seen an explosion of information available from specialist sites.

All of this means that there are three main groups of information resources available to those with an internet connection:

- databases
- specialist websites
- secondary journals.

Databases

Here we outline a range of useful databases for those interested in evidence-based practice. Access arrangements to these vary in different countries. In the UK, access is either available free or to NHS staff using an Athens password.

Cochrane Library

The *Cochrane Library* is published on a quarterly basis and contains a number of databases:

- Cochrane Database of Systematic Reviews
- Database of Abstracts of Reviews of Effects (DARE)
- Cochrane Central Register of Controlled Trials (CENTRAL)
- Cochrane Methodology Register
- NHS Economic Evaluation Database
- Health Technology Assessment Database
- Cochrane Database of Methodology Reviews (CDMR).

Cochrane Database of Systematic Reviews

This contains all the systematic reviews published by the Cochrane Collaboration and the protocols of all the systematic reviews that are currently in preparation. Cochrane reviews are some of the most methodologically rigorous reviews conducted and are kept under regular review.

Database of Abstracts of Reviews of Effects (DARE)

DARE is produced by the Centre for Reviews and Dissemination at the University of York and contains structured abstracts of non-Cochrane reviews that have been quality assessed.

Cochrane Central Register of Controlled Trials (CENTRAL)
This is a database of definitive controlled trials that has been established by contributors to the Cochrane Collaboration and others, as part of an international effort to identify all clinical trials, as existing bibliographic databases are inadequate to identify all trials. The Cochrane Collaboration embarked upon this formidable task in cooperation with the National Library of Medicine (NLM) in Washington, DC (USA), which produces MEDLINE, and Reed Elsevier of Amsterdam (the Netherlands) which produces EMBASE. There are currently over 300,000 records in the database.

Cochrane Methodology Register
The *Cochrane Methodology Register* (CMR) is a database of studies relevant to the methods of systematic reviews of healthcare and social interventions. The register includes journal articles, book chapters, conference proceedings, conference abstracts and reports of ongoing methodological research. The register aims to include all published reports of empirical methodological studies that could be relevant for inclusion in a Cochrane methodology review, along with comparative and descriptive studies relevant to the conduct of systematic reviews of healthcare interventions. In Issue 2, 2006, of the *Cochrane Library*, CMR contains 8255 records.

The NHS Economic Evaluation Database
The NHS Economic Evaluation Database (NHS EED) project is commissioned by the NHS Research and Development Programme to identify as many studies as possible on economic evaluations in the literature and to disseminate the principal findings to clinicians and other decision makers by means of structured and critical abstracts. The abstracts are freely accessible through a public database on the internet (available through www.york.ac.uk/inst/crd) and also from the *Cochrane Library*. The aim of the project is to assist researchers and decision makers in identifying and interpreting economic evaluations, which are spread over many databases and paper-based resources.

The database currently holds 1800 structured abstracts of full economic evaluations (cost-effectiveness, cost utility, and cost–benefit studies) and bibliographic details of 1953 cost studies, 649 reviews (of cost-effectiveness), and 459 studies of methodology.

Health Technology Assessment (HTA) database
See www.york.ac.uk/inst/crd/crddatabases.htm
The HTA database is produced by the Centre for Reviews and Dissemination in collaboration with the secretariat of INAHTA (International Network of

Agencies for Health Technology Assessment). This database contains details of nearly 5000 completed HTA publications and around 800 ongoing INAHTA projects.

Cochrane Database of Methodology Reviews

This is a specific collection of records of reports and empirical studies relating to the methods of systematic reviews and the evaluation of health and social care more generally. The register contains information for several thousand reports, and prospective entries for ongoing methodological research.

Other Databases

PubMed

PubMed (www.pubmed.gov) was developed by the National Center for Biotechnology Information (NCBI) at the National Library of Medicine (NLM), located at the US National Institutes of Health (NIH). PubMed provides access to bibliographic information that includes MEDLINE and OLDMEDLINE.

MEDLINE

MEDLINE is the NLM's premier bibliographic database covering the fields of medicine, nursing, dentistry, veterinary medicine, the healthcare system and the preclinical sciences. MEDLINE contains more than 4800 biomedical journals published in the United States and 70 other countries. The database contains over 14 million citations dating back to the mid-1960s. Coverage is worldwide but most records are from English-language sources or have English abstracts.

OLDMEDLINE

OLDMEDLINE currently contains approximately 2 million citations to articles from international biomedical journals from 1950 through 1965. NLM expects to continue converting citations from its older print medical indexes and to add these citations to PubMed. OLDMEDLINE citations do not include abstracts.

EMBASE

EMBASE from Elsevier B.V. is a pharmacological and biomedical database with extensive indexing of drug information from 4550 journals published in 70 countries. More than 80% of the records contain abstracts. The database includes EMTREE, a hierarchically ordered controlled thesaurus, which contains 46,000 preferred terms and more than 200,000 synonyms.

PsycINFO (formally Psychlit)
PsycINFO is a database that provides abstracts and citations to the scholarly literature in the behavioural sciences and mental health from the 1800s to the present. It includes material of relevance to psychologists and professionals in related fields such as psychiatry, management, business, education, social science, neuroscience, law, medicine and social work.

CINHAL
CINAHL, the Cumulative Index to Nursing and Allied Health Literature, is a database providing coverage of the professional literature in nursing and 17 allied health disciplines and also covers consumer health, biomedicine, alternative therapy, and health sciences librarianship. The database has over 545,000 records, with coverage from 1982 to the present, and is updated monthly.

LILACS
LILACS indexes the regional literature from Latin America and the Caribbean. It includes over 670 journals (only 41 overlap with MEDLINE/EMBASE) with abstracts in English, Portuguese or Spanish. It uses MEDLINE's medical subject headings (MeSH) and is edited by BIREME (Latin American and Caribbean Center on Health Science Information, www.bireme.br). BIREME is an agency of the Pan-American Health Organization/World Health Organization.

SciELO
The Scientific Electronic Library Online is a model for cooperative electronic publishing of scientific journals on the internet. Conceived to meet the scientific communication needs of developing countries, particularly Latin America and the Caribbean countries, it provides an efficient way to assure universal visibility and accessibility to their scientific literature.

SciELO is the product of a partnership between FAPESP (the State of São Paulo Science Foundation, www.fapesp.br), BIREME (the Latin American and Caribbean Center on Health Sciences Information, www.bireme.br), as well as national and international institutions related to scientific communication and editors. Since 2002, the Project has also been supported by CNPq (Conselho Nacional de Desenvolvimento Científico e Tecnológico, www.cnpq.br).

Specialist Websites
The evidence-based approach has seen a number of specialist websites develop to help support those interested in the approach and provide information.

The Centre for Evidence-based Dentistry
The Centre for Evidence-based Dentistry website (www.cebd.org) is one of the oldest evidence-based dentistry sites, having been established in 1998. It provides links to a wide range of resources to support the practice of EBD and topic-based links to high-quality evidence. It also has links to most of the useful available evidence-based dentistry resources on the web.

Cochrane Oral Health Group
The Cochrane Oral Health Group website (www.ohg.cochrane.org) provides links to all the abstracts of all the Cochrane reviews conducted by the Oral Health Group, protocols and titles of reviews under consideration. It also has details of how to join the group and details of its activity.

Oral Health Specialist Library (OHSL)
The Oral Health Specialist Library (www.library.nhs.uk/oralhealth) is one of the branch libraries of the National Library for Health (NLH). The NLH provides a wide range of high-quality resources for clinicians, a significant proportion of which is freely available. However, to access some elements of the site (e.g. online journal and databases), an Athens password is required.

The OHSL is a developing resource providing summaries of high-quality information for clinicians as well as links to a range of evidence-based resources. The quality control on this site is high so users can use the information safely. All the core content provided on the OHSL is free.

Pan American Centers for Evidence Based Dentistry
This new website (www.evidentista.org) was launched in September 2006. It has been developed by a number of collaborators with seed funding from the International Association of Dental Research and the Fulbright Scholar Program and is available in English, Spanish and Portuguese. One of its key features is a clinical question-and-answer section with a short, direct answer to the clinical question with links to more details.

Secondary Journals
Secondary journals have developed with evidence-based practice. Most have similar operating models in that they sift through the wide range of material available in other journals, selecting the better articles and producing summaries of the original articles together with commentaries from experts in the field. This greatly reduces the number of articles individual dentists need to read in order to keep up to date. There are two dental journals produced in this way, *Evidence-based Dentistry* and *Evidence-based Dental Practice*.

Table A-1 **Search strategy to find the best type of restoration for carious primary molar teeth** (continued)

Search	Query	Result
10.	stainless steel crown	544
11.	preformed metal crowns	46
12.	"Crowns" [MeSH]	11,417
13.	#1 OR #2 OR #3 OR #4 OR #5 OR #6 OR #7 OR #8 OR #9 OR #10 OR #11 OR #12	11,439
14.	Pain	338,842
15.	"Pain" [MeSH]	204,098
16.	swelling	65,294
17.	survival	590,401
18.	"Survival Rate" [MeSH] OR "Survival Analysis" [MeSH]	139,383
19.	tooth loss	2270
20.	"Tooth Loss" [MeSH]	1486
21.	#14 OR #15 OR #16 OR #17 OR #18 OR #19 OR #20	597,076
22.	#13 AND #21	318
23.	"Tooth, Deciduous" [MeSH]	7435
24.	primary teeth	8024
25.	#23 OR #24	8024
26.	#25 AND #22	16

Finding the Best Method of Preventing Root Caries in Adults

Question	Patient	Intervention	Comparison	Outcome
What is the best method of preventing root caries in adult patients?	Adult at risk of root caries	Topical fluorides, restorations, diet modification, chlorhexidine mouthwash	Topical fluorides, restorations, diet modification, chlorhexidine mouthwash	Caries

Table A-2 **Search strategy to find the best method of preventing root caries in adults**

Search	Query	Result
1.	root caries	768
2.	"Root Caries" [MeSH]	495
3.	#1 OR #2	768
4.	topical fluoride	3776
5.	"Fluorides, Topical" [MeSH]	3339
6.	Diet	24,5001
7.	"Food Habits" [MeSH]	11,634
8.	tooth restoration	9085
9.	"Dental Restoration, Permanent" [MeSH]	27,717
10.	chlorhexidine	5070
11.	"Chlorhexidine" [MeSH]	4011
12.	#4 OR #5 OR #6 OR #7 OR #8 OR #9 OR #10 OR #11	288,570
13.	#3 AND #12	283
14.	(systematic[sb]) OR (meta-analysis) OR (metaanalysis) OR (systematic review)*	1,290,456
15.	#13 AND #14	49

* represents a specific short search strategy to identify systematic reviews

Finding the Side-effects of Chlorhexidine Mouthwash for the Treatment of Periodontal Disease

Question	Patient	Intervention	Comparison	Outcome
What are the side-effects of using chlorhexidine mouthwash for the treatment of periodontal disease?	Adults with perio-dontal disease	Chlorhexidine mouthwash	Placebo	Staining, altered taste

Table A-3 **Search strategy to find the side-effects of using chlorhexidine mouthwash for the treatment of periodontal disease**

Search	Query	Result
1.	periodon*	56,057
2.	"Periodontal Diseases" [MeSH]	49,323
3.	#1 OR #2	69,645
4.	chlorhexidine mouthwash	4105
5.	"Chlorhexidine" [MeSH]	4011
6.	#4 OR #5	4105
7.	side effects	1,235,066
8.	adverse effects	1,198,084
9.	"adverse effects" [Subheading]	1,173,441
10.	#7 OR #8 OR #9	1,258,176
11.	#3 AND #6	1001
12.	#10 AND #11	190
13.	(systematic[sb]) OR (meta-analysis) OR (metaanalysis) OR (systematic review)*	1,290,456
14.	#12 AND #13	27

* is the symbol for a truncation, i.e. the database is searched for all words beginning with periodon: periodontal, periodontitis, Periodontology etc.

To Discover if Digital X-rays are Better at Diagnosing Caries than Film-based Systems

Question	Patient	Intervention	Comparison	Outcome
Are digital x-ray systems better at diagnosing caries than film-based systems?	All patients requiring dental x-rays	Digital x-ray	Film-based x-ray systems	Improved diagnosis, increased sensitivity and specificity

Table A-4 **Search strategy to discover if digital x-ray systems are better at diagnosing caries than film-based systems**

Search	Query	Result
1.	caries	34,640
2.	"Dental Caries" [MeSH]	29,194
3.	#1 OR #2	
4.	dental radiography	12,623
5.	"Radiography, Dental" [MeSH]	12,573
6.	digital radiograph^	1275
7.	"Radiography, Dental, Digital" [MeSH]	775
8.	#4 OR #5 OR #6 OR #7	13,623
9.	#3 AND #8	830
10.	sensitivity	520,141
11.	specificity	587,760
12.	#10 AND #11	253,775
13.	"Sensitivity and Specificity" [MeSH]	211,637
14.	#12 OR #14	253,775
15.	#9 AND #14	221
16.	(systematic[sb]) OR (meta-analysis) OR (metaanalysis) OR (systematic review)	1,290,456
17.	#15 AND #16	17

To Discover if School-based Toothbrushing Programmes are Cost-effective

Question	Patient	Intervention	Comparison	Outcome
Are school-based tooth-brushing programmes cost-effective?	School-aged children	Toothbrushing programmes	No programme	Cost effec-tiveness

Table A-5 **Search strategy to discover if school-based toothbrushing programmes are cost-effective**

Search	Query	Result
1.	toothbrushing	4819
2.	"Toothbrushing" [MeSH]	4433
3.	#1 OR #2	4819
4.	school	139,428
5.	"Schools" [MeSH]	52,835
6.	#4 OR #5	139,428
7.	#3 AND #6	437
8.	cost effectiveness	45,946
9.	cost benefit	40,945
10.	cost minimisation	152
11.	"Cost-Benefit Analysis" [MeSH]	38,480
12.	"Costs and Cost Analysis" [MeSH]	124,612
13.	#8 OR #9 OR #10 OR #11 OR #12	132,834
14.	#13 AND #7	8

To Find What Teenagers' Reasons are for Undergoing Orthodontic Treatment

Question	Patient	Intervention	Comparison	Outcome
What are teenagers' reasons for undergoing orthodontic treatment?	Children requiring orthodontic treatment	Orthodontic treatment		Improved compliance

Table A-6 **Search strategy to find what teenagers' reasons are for undergoing orthodontic treatment**

Search	Query	Result
1.	orthodont*	36,666
2.	"Orthodontics" [MeSH]	31,391
3.	#1 OR #2	39,666
4.	compliance	73,241
5.	"Patient Compliance" [MeSH]	29,810
6.	reasons for undergoing	1606
7.	Patient Participation	11,178
8.	"Patient Acceptance of Health Care" [MeSH]	90,737
9.	#4 OR #5 OR #6 OR #7 OR #8 OR #9	134,756
10.	#3 AND #9	961
11.	teenager	1,145,662
12.	"Adolescent" [MeSH]	1,143,089
13.	#10 OR #11	1,145,662
14.	#10 AND #13	402
15.	questionnaire	212,663
16.	interview	83,503
17.	focus group	7972
18.	#15 OR #16 OR #17	282,067
19.	#14 AND #18	105

Answer to Exercise on Page 98

Calculating Sensitivity, Specificity, Positive and Negative Predictive Values and Likelihood Ratio

	Reference standard		
	Disease present	Disease absent	
Test positive	215 a	b 16	231 $(a + b)$
Test negative	15 c	d 114	129 $(c + d)$
Total	230 $(a + c)$	130 $(b + d)$	360 $(a + b + c + d)$

Sensitivity (detection rate) $= \dfrac{\text{All those with the disease who test positive}}{\text{All those with the disease}}$

$$= \frac{a}{a + c} = \frac{215}{230}$$

$$= 0.9347 = 93.5\%$$

Specificity $= \dfrac{\text{All those who test negative who don't have the disease}}{\text{All those without the disease}}$

$$= \frac{d}{b + d} = \frac{114}{130}$$

$$= 0.8769 = 87.7\%$$

Positive predictive value $= \dfrac{\text{All those with the disease who test positive}}{\text{All those with a positive test}}$

$$= \frac{a}{a + b} = \frac{215}{231}$$

$$= 0.9307 = 93\%$$

$$\text{Negative predictive value} = \frac{\text{All those without the disease who test negative}}{\text{All those with a negative test}}$$

$$= \frac{d}{c + d} = \frac{114}{129}$$

$$= 0.8837 = 88.4\%$$

$$\text{LR} = \frac{\text{Sensitivity}}{(1 - \text{Specificity})}$$

$$= \frac{0.9347}{1 - 0.8769}$$

$$= 7.593$$

Glossary

Alpha/beta errors

Alpha (Type I) errors are false positives; that is, the results suggest that a treatment works, when in fact it does not work. Beta (Type II) errors are false negatives; that is, the results suggest a treatment does not work, when in fact it actually does.

Association

A known link, or statistical dependence, between two or more conditions or variables; for example, statistics demonstrate that there is an association between smoking and lung cancer.

Beta errors

See entry for *Alpha/beta errors*.

Bias

Something that introduces a difference or trend that distorts (or could distort) results of a study.

Blind(ed) study

Study where the observer(s) and/or participants are kept ignorant of the group to which the participants are assigned. Where both observer and participants are kept ignorant, the study is termed double-blind. If the statistical analysis is also done blind the study is triple-blind. The purpose of blinding is to remove bias.

Case–control study

Compares people with a disease or condition ("cases") with another group of people from the same population who do not have that disease or condition ("controls"). A case–control study can identify risks and trends and suggest some possible causes for disease, or for particular outcomes.

Case-series

A report on a series of patients with an outcome of interest. No control group is involved.

Cochrane Collaboration

The Cochrane Collaboration is an international effort by researchers, practitioners and consumers to sift through research on the effects of healthcare. The Collaboration prepares, maintains and disseminates systematic reviews of the effects of healthcare. The reviews are published in the Cochrane Database of Systematic Reviews, one of the components of the Cochrane Library.

Cohort (study)

A cohort is a group of people clearly identified; a cohort study follows that group over time and reports on what happens to them. A cohort study is an observational study and it can be prospective or retrospective.

Confidence interval (CI)

Confidence interval is the range within which the true size of effect (never exactly known) lies with a given degree of assurance. People often speak of a "95% confidence interval" (or "95% confidence limits"). This is the interval which includes the true value in 95% of cases.

Confounding variable

A variable that is not the one you are interested in but which may affect the results of the trial.

Cross-over trial

A trial where each of the groups will receive each of the treatments, but in a randomised order: that is, they will start off in one arm of the trial, but will deliberately cross over to the other arm(s) in turn.

Cross-sectional study

Also called prevalence study. An observational study, taking a view of a group of people at one point in time and seeing the prevalence of diseases, for example, in that population.

Decision analysis

The application of explicit, quantitative methods to analyse decisions under conditions of uncertainty.

Ecological survey

A study based on aggregated data for some population as it exists at some point in time; to investigate the relationship of an exposure to a known or presumed risk factor for a specific outcome.

Effectiveness (clinical effectiveness)

The extent to which an intervention does people more good than harm. An effective treatment or intervention is effective in real-life circumstances, not just an ideal situation.

Efficacy

The extent to which an intervention improves the outcome for people under ideal circumstances. Testing efficacy means finding out whether something is capable of causing an effect at all.

Heterogeneous/heterogeneity

The opposite of homogeneous. If a set of studies on the same subject have varied or conflicting results, the results of the group of studies are heterogeneous. Examining and explaining this heterogeneity is an important part of reviewing the research on a particular subject.

Incidence

The number of occurrences of something in a population over a particular period of time, e.g. the number of cases of a disease in a country over one year.

Intent(ion)-to-treat analysis

Analysing the results according to the intended treatment to which someone was allocated in a randomised controlled trial (as opposed to the treatment they actually received in the end).

Meta-analysis

Meta-analysis is a statistical technique which summarises the results of several studies into a single estimate, giving more weight to results from larger studies.

Number needed to treat (NNT)

One measure of a treatment's clinical effectiveness. It is the number of people you would need to treat with a specific intervention (e.g. aspirin for people having a heart attack) to see one occurrence of a specific outcome (e.g. prevention of death).

Odds

A term little used outside gambling and statistics. It is defined as the ratio of the probability of an event happening, to that of its not happening: the risk.

Odds ratio (OR)

One measure of a treatment's clinical effectiveness. If the OR = 1 then the effects of the treatment are no different from those of the control treatment. If the OR is greater (or less) than 1 then the effects of the treatment are more (or less) than those of the control treatment. Note that the effects being measured may be adverse (e.g. death, disability) or desirable (e.g. stopping smoking).

Power (statistical power)

A study needs to have a specific level of power in order to be able to reliably detect a difference that a treatment might cause. The study needs to have enough participants, who experience enough of the outcomes in question, to be able to come up with statistically significant results.

Prevalence

The proportion of a population having a particular condition or characteristic, e.g. the percentage of people in a city with a particular disease, or who smoke.

Probability

Probability is the chance or risk of something happening (see also the entry for *p*-value below).

Probability (*p*-)value

The findings of a study may be just an unusual fluke. Calculating the *p*-value can determine whether or not the results of the study are likely to be a fluke. The *p* (probability) value shows whether or not the result could have been caused by chance. If the *p*-value is less than 0.05, then the result is not due to chance. A result with a *p*-value of less than 0.05 is statistically significant. The 0.05 level is equal to odds of 19 to 1 (or a 1 in 20 chance).
(See also entries for *Confidence interval*, *Power* and *Probability*.)

Publication bias

A bias in a systematic review caused by incompleteness of a search, such as omitting non-English language sources or unpublished trials (inconclusive trails are less likely to be published than conclusive ones but are not necessarily less valid).

Quasi-random

Methods of allocating people to a trial which are not strictly random, e.g. allocation by the person's date of birth, the day of the week, by medical record number, or just allocating every alternate person. Quasi-random allocation may look random but in fact it is not because the group to which a person will be allocated is predictable and thus people can manipulate who enters the group. For example, if someone wants to be in the experimental group, but not the control group, they can be placed in the experimental group if their number has come up, and simply excluded from the trial if it doesn't. One, other or both arms of the trial can then be biased. (See also the entry for *Randomised controlled trial* below.)

Randomised controlled trial (RCT)

An RCT is a trial in which subjects are randomly assigned to two groups: one (the experimental group) receiving the intervention that is being tested, and the other (the comparison group or controls) receiving an alternative treatment. The two groups are then followed up to see if any differences between them result. This helps people assess the effectiveness of the intervention.

Relative risk (RR)

Also called the risk ratio, the RR is a common way of estimating the risk of experiencing a particular effect or result. An RR >1 means a person is estimated to be at an increased risk, while an RR <1 means a person is apparently at decreased risk. An RR of 1.0 means there is no apparent effect on risk at all. For example, if the RR = 4.0, the result is about 4 times more likely to happen, and 0.25 means it is 4 times less likely to happen. (See also entries for *Confidence interval* and *Odds ratio*.)

Risk difference

Also called absolute risk reduction. It is literally the difference in size of risk between two groups. For example, if one group has a 15% incidence of a disease, and the other has a 10% incidence of the disease, the risk difference is 5%.

Sensitivity analysis

A process of testing how sensitive a result would be to changes in the factors such as baseline risk, susceptibility or the patients' best and worst outcome.

Spectrum bias

A bias caused by a study population whose disease profile does not reflect that of the intended population (e.g. if they have more severe forms of the disorder).

Standard deviation

A set measure of how far things vary from the central result (average). The mean is the central (average) measure. The standard deviation (SD) is a way of describing how far away from this centre, or average, the values spread. For example, a mean waiting time in a hospital emergency room might be 2 hours, but to cover most people's waiting time, you might have to give or take an hour: the waiting time is therefore 2 ± 1 hours. That extra 1 hour is the standard deviation. A person who waited 4 hours to be seen would therefore be 2 SD from the mean.

Statistical significance

The findings of a study may be just an unusual fluke. A statistical test can determine whether or not the results of the study are likely to be a fluke. That test calculates the probability of the result being caused by chance, providing a probability (*p*) value.

Systematic review

A review in which evidence on a topic has been systematically identified, appraised and summarised according to predetermined criteria (an "overview").

Validity

The soundness or rigour of a study. A study is valid if the way it is designed and carried out means that the results are unbiased, i.e. it gives you a true estimate of clinical effectiveness.

Index

Quintessentials for General Dental Practitioners Series

in 44 volumes

Editor-in-Chief: Professor Nairn H F Wilson

The Quintessentials for General Dental Practitioners Series covers basic principles and key issues in all aspects of modern dental medicine. Each book can be read as a stand-alone volume or in conjunction with other books in the series.

	Publication date, approximately
Clinical Practice, Editor: Nairn Wilson	
Culturally Sensitive Oral Healthcare	available
Dental Erosion	available
Special Care Dentistry	available
Evidence-based Dentistry	available
Infection Control for the Dental Team	Summer 2008
Oral Surgery and Oral Medicine, Editor: John G Meechan	
Practical Dental Local Anaesthesia	available
Practical Oral Medicine	available
Practical Conscious Sedation	available
Minor Oral Surgery in Dental Practice	available
Imaging, Editor: Keith Horner	
Interpreting Dental Radiographs	available
Panoramic Radiology	available
21st Century Dental Imaging	available
Periodontology, Editor: Iain L C Chapple	
Understanding Periodontal Diseases: Assessment and Diagnostic Procedures in Practice	available
Decision-Making for the Periodontal Team	available
Successful Periodontal Therapy – A Non-Surgical Approach	available
Periodontal Management of Children, Adolescents and Young Adults	available
Periodontal Medicine: A Window on the Body	available
Contemporary Periodontal Surgery – An Illustrated Guide to the Art Behind the Science	available